FIRST, BOB PARIS TOOK YOU

BEYOND BUILT

"THIS BOOK IS PRICELESS. Contains secrets on how a man, any man, not just a bodybuilder, can achieve his ideal body—and it's easy to follow. Bob gives away secrets."

> —**Joyce Vedral,** author of
> *The Fat-Burning Workout*
> and *Gut Busters*

"LISTEN TO WHAT HE HAS TO SAY. IT CAN HELP YOU CREATE YOUR IDEAL WORKOUT. Bob Paris is a great bodybuilding champion who knows the ins and outs of creating a muscular physique."

> —**Joe Weider,** publisher of
> *Muscle and Fitness, Shape, Flex,*
> and *Men's Fitness* magazines

"*BEYOND BUILT*'S WELL-ROUNDED APPROACH TAKES THE BUNK OUT OF BUILDING AN OUTSTANDING PHYSIQUE."

> —**Lee Labrada,**
> IFBB World Champion
> and Mr. Olympia Finalist

"BOB'S WORK SHINES. His exercise content, description and evaluation are outstanding. Few pros succeed in explaining exercise movement and muscle performance as effectively and clearly...Bob's mastery is evident."
> —**Dave Draper**

"LEARNING FROM A CHAMPION LIKE BOB WILL MAXIMIZE YOUR POTENTIAL... *BEYOND BUILT* will thoroughly educate you, and provide a complete understanding of bodybuilding's most important elements."
> —**Lou Ferrigno**

NOW, LET HIM MAKE YOU

FLAWLESS

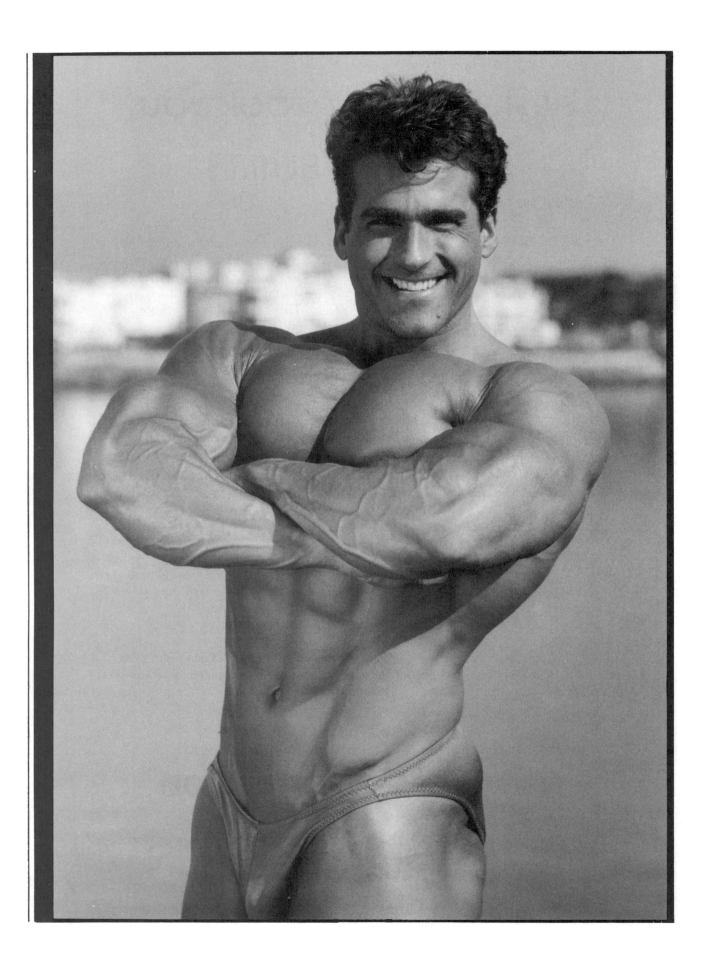

FLAWLESS

THE TEN-WEEK, TOTAL-IMAGE METHOD FOR
TRANSFORMING YOUR PHYSIQUE

BOB PARIS

WARNER BOOKS

A Time Warner Company

To Rod, with all my love.
Your heart and spirit are my life's anchor.
I can only hope that I am one-one-millionth as "Flawless"
in your eyes and heart as you are in mine.

The information in the book reflects the author's experiences and is not intended to replace medical advice. Any questions regarding your individual health, general or specific, should be addressed to your physician.

Before beginning this or any other exercise or nutritional regimen, consult your physician to be sure it is appropriate for you.

A portion of Bob Jackson-Paris's royalties from *Flawless* will benefit the American Foundation for AIDS Research and the Be True To Yourself Foundation.

Copyright © 1993 by Bob Paris
All rights reserved.

Warner Books, Inc., 1271 Avenue of the Americas, New York, NY 10020
 A Time Warner Company

Printed in the United States of America
First Printing: March 1993
10 9 8 7 6 5

Library of Congress Cataloging-in-Publication Data
Paris, Bob.
   Flawless : the ten-week, total-image method for transforming your physique / Bob Paris.
      p.   cm.
   Includes index.
   ISBN 0-446-39406-8
   1. Bodybuilding—Training.   I. Title.
GV546.P265   1993
646.7'5—dc20   92-26768
                                                         CIP

Cover design by Diane Luger
Cover photo by Robert Reiff
Book design by Giorgetta Bell McRee

ACKNOWLEDGMENTS

I'd like to take a moment to thank several people who either contributed to the creation of this book or who have influenced my views on fitness and bodybuilding.

First, many thanks to my editor, Rick Horgan, whose patience and prodding helped take the project from development to completion.

Another important contributor was my good friend Art Zeller. His master photographer's skill has once again exceeded itself in the work that illustrates this book. Bravo, Artie.

Thanks also to photographer Robert Rieff for his photo contributions. They were very much appreciated.

I'd like to voice my gratitude to Joe and Ben Weider for their tireless work in the advancement and promotion of bodybuilding and fitness.

Much gratitude also to Robert Kennedy, Tom Deters, Jim Rosenthal, Jerry Kindela, Jim Chada, John Balik and the many other editors and publishers whose editorial support helped make my previous book, *Beyond Built*, a success, thereby making room for *Flawless.*

CONTENTS

AUTHOR'S NOTE

> "Whatever you can do, or dream you can, begin it. Boldness has genius, power and magic to it."
>
> —GOETHE

Dear Reader:

This book is intended both as an adjunct to my first book, *Beyond Built*, and as an independent volume that can be fully appreciated apart from the previous work.

If you were a reader of *Beyond Built*, welcome to what could be regarded as "a step beyond." That's where we'll venture in the next few hundred pages: beyond the basics, and beyond abstract philosophy into a program that will definitely transform your body during an intense ten-week period.

Make no mistake about it, this book is about work. It will take work and commitment on your part to make the transformation to "flawlessness" in only ten weeks.

Since, however, the work involved will lead directly to self-improvement, you'll find yourself eagerly looking forward to the next workout. As each week passes you'll feel an enhanced sense of achievement. And, vicariously at least, I'll be sharing in your excitement.

One of my greatest pleasures in life is to watch as someone discovers the tremendous benefits that can come from a well-planned, goal-oriented fitness, nutrition and self-improvement program.

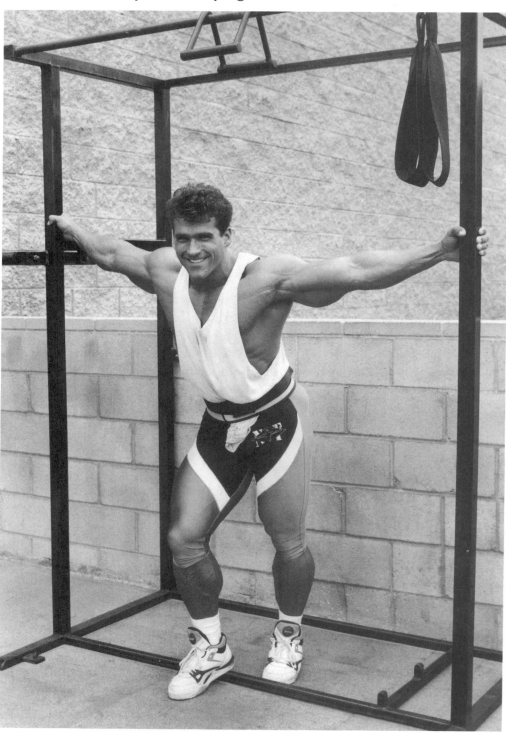

INTRODUCTION

What is the overall purpose of this book? The answer is fairly simple and at the same time rather complex. The simple answer is that I've written this book to provide a direct, no-nonsense, step-by-step method for achieving the greatest possible transformation over the next ten weeks. And, of course, you are looking for the secret of how this transformation can be accomplished. The complex part of the answer lies in motivation. What is it that motivates you to want to make this dramatic change? It could be any of thousands of reasons. I can think of several right off the top of my head.

Perhaps you've just learned that you have a high school reunion coming up and you want to show up looking great. Or it may be the middle of spring and despite that New Year's resolution, you still have an extra ten pounds bulging indiscreetly in all the wrong places. You definitely want to whip yourself into shape in time for your first beach weekend on Memorial Day, ten weeks away. Or how about this one? You've just stopped smoking and can't believe the shape you've let yourself get into. The health insurance company's required physical is ten weeks away and your doctor says if you don't pull yourself together you might very well be canceled—your policy *and* you. Sound rough? It is. Some people need major alarm clocks to go off before they begin to take action. Ask someone recovering from a heart attack how much more precious life is to them now.

So let's narrow the basic motivations down to two. Health, and...well, let's be honest: vanity.

You might be saying, "Well, I see what you mean by health, but this vanity business—that just doesn't fit me at all." Right.

The thing is, vanity is not necessarily a bad thing. The word itself just happens to be loaded with a lot of negative connotations: conceit, selfishness, etc.

That's not the "vanity" I'm talking about. I'm talking about being interested enough in your own appearance and well-being to put forth an effort to create positive change and maintain it until the next change needs to be made. So maybe you'd be more comfortable if instead of using the word "vanity," I substituted "self-esteem."

Throughout this book I'll be talking about changes that will have a dramatic effect on your self-esteem. I don't care how high your self-esteem is at this moment, it can always improve. It's not like you're trying to fill a gallon jug with water and only so much will fit before it's full. There is no upper limit to how good you can feel about yourself and your appearance. So dare yourself to make the change.

After all, one of the only constant things in life is change. If you're not moving in a positive direction, you're moving in a negative one. Even the failure to take positive action will result in negative consequences. You know the old sayings:

"You are what you eat."

"Take care of your body and it will take care of you."

"A mind is a terrible thing to waste."

And so on.

We live in a society that puts a great deal of emphasis on physical appearance. The approach I want you to take goes a few steps beyond surface beauty. Of course, the appearance of your body is very important, but it doesn't tell the whole story. To be truly "flawless" you need to combine the look you desire—and are willing to invest in achieving—with healthy inner workings. So what I will help you pursue will be *whole body fitness.* The training and nutrition routines I've developed will reflect that emphasis.

What I'm asking you to do is to make an investment in yourself. When it comes right down to it, *you* are all you really have in life. Oh, you might have a lot of material things...but things can be taken away or forgotten. If you don't believe me, think back to something you couldn't live without as a kid. Maybe it was a bike. As time went on, this bike that you couldn't live without was probably forgotten, sold, lost, stolen or passed on to someone else who couldn't live without it. You, however, were still right there. Right in the center of your own life. My point is, no matter what, you always have yourself to make an investment in. I don't care how old you are, how out of shape or unathletic you may now consider yourself to be. You can begin from this moment on to make a positive investment in your future.

Give yourself the chance to break away from where you are now. If you've never exercised before, open yourself up to discovering the incredible benefits that can come from taking control of your health and physical appearance. If you're experienced in the gym, give yourself a chance to break through to a new level of development and achievement. A ten-week commitment is all I'm asking.

It's up to you to decide how badly you want it. Do you want to be flawless so much that it hurts? Have you been talking forever about making the changes that will make you proud of your body? Now is the time to take action on that dream of yours. I'm here to show you how to make it a reality.

Let's talk for a moment about visualization. Does the term "visualization" give you a weird feeling? For some the word conjures up visions (no pun intended) of some sort of woo-woo new-age mysticism. For others it means a talent that someone possesses innately.

Many people are skeptical of visualization techniques because they've been asked somewhere along the line to close their eyes and visualize this or that. When they did and a Technicolor, 3-D, Dolby-stereo epic feature didn't immediately begin, they got frustrated and gave up.

Visualization is neither a religious ritual nor a magical ability possessed by a chosen few. It is a skill (similar to weight training, bowling or writing your name) that must be developed through practice. Of course, it's also helpful to understand just what that skill is. The dictionary definition of visualization is, "formation of mental visual images." Depending on the person, this image can be a still picture, a movie, something that is clear and in focus, something that is fuzzy and out of focus, a scene in black and white or in color. Some people's mental images are formed by internal dialogue—a sort of running commentary describing the image's various elements. Still others get "a sense" of their mental images—not quite a picture, but not really words either. Most of us have bits of each of these pictures, word and sense categories playing in our imagination, but one is usually dominant.

I mentioned that visualization is a skill similar to learning to write your name. When you were a kid and learning to write your name, you probably thought that you would never master this monumental task that all big people took so much for granted. But you did, and then used the same technique to master many other skills as the years went on. The technique is rehearsal and repetition.

Through rehearsal and repetition, visualization can become a powerful tool in helping to turn your dreams into reality. These days almost all top athletes use mental rehearsal and visualization techniques to bolster their physical performances.

The mental workouts to develop these skills will be included in the training sections that follow. For the next five minutes, though, I'd like you to put this book aside and vividly imagine yourself having achieved your wildest dream. The dream can be big or small, relate to physical development or general life success. The point is, it must be packed with meaning for you. Please try to use all five senses to imagine yourself in the middle of this fantasy-come-true...

> "Whatever the mind...can conceive and believe it can achieve."
> —NAPOLEON HILL

All right, it's five minutes later. How do you feel? Extremely upbeat, positive and energetic, I would imagine. Do you know why? Because vividly imagining your dreams starts the physical, chemical and emotional process that can lead to goal achievement. The only missing element is the action. Action is required to go beyond the vision and develop a successful result.

What we need to do is separate those dreams that we only want to visualize from the ones that we want to act on. As you can see, "action" is the key word here. It's going to take the action of getting up, making the commitment and following through for you to achieve a flawless body.

Just what is a flawless body? Do you have to look like a Mr. America to be flawless? Absolutely not...not unless your goal is to be a Mr. America. Do you have to look like an Olympic gymnast to be flawless? Absolutely not ...not unless your goal is to be or look like a world-class gymnast. You see, flawlessness is different for every person. My own definition of "flawlessness" has meaning for everybody regardless of body type and goal level. The recipe for achieving a flawless body is made of the following elements:

1. Dreams—Your hopes and aspirations. It's vital to separate those dreams that you want to act on from those that will only remain fanciful clouds.

2. Desire—A dream taken to the point where you ask yourself to act on it.

3. Reality—Acknowledging your unique circumstances. In developing a workout program, you must take into account *your* bone structure, metabolism, muscle structure, motivation and ability to follow through.

4. Goals—A desire combined with a strategy for attaining the outcome that you will work toward.

5. Work—The physical and mental effort put toward attaining a goal. The willingness to put forth that effort.

6. Enthusiasm—A passionate interest in doing the work that will accomplish the desired goal.

7. Perseverance—The ability to keep going even when there is no light at the end of the tunnel.

8. Patience—The ability to realize that no goal will be accomplished instantly. Being able to put in all the work and to wait calmly for the desired outcome.

9. Experience—Becoming skilled at a task by action and observation. The knowledge gained by working toward an outcome.

10. Flexibility—The ability to know when something is not working and to make a strategic change. Flexibility does not override persistence, but it is rooted in reality and patience.

When it comes down to it, a "flawless" body is the body you envision as being perfect for you. There are two elements, though, that I think must be present regardless of individual perspective.

The first is balanced muscle development. Even if you don't want big legs, you should train them anyway. To me, nothing looks funnier than a completely unbalanced body. For example, I have seen swimsuit ads where the model appeared to have worked chest and abdominals very hard, but the legs had obviously never been touched. To me this is a funny look. You should go after full-body fitness, not just the spot fitness that happens when you focus on one or two body parts. (In later chapters, I'll explain why balanced training is far more than just aesthetically pleasing.)

The second element is a low level of body fat. Am I talking about the ultra low levels that physique athletes have on contest day? No, not unless your body naturally maintains that level of body fat on a year-round basis. (If your ten-week goal for this program is to peak as a bodybuilder, then you would of course be an exception.)

What most people don't understand, though, is that for almost all competitive bodybuilders, that ultralow body-fat level is temporary. It's a goal the athlete works toward, understanding that it will not last. The photos that you see in a physique magazine are almost always taken around competition time, when the athlete is close to peak condition (highest level of muscle mass and lowest level of body fat). We are not talking about a "real world" situation. So your body-fat levels must be determined by your own unique metabolism and structure. The level should be low for your body. It should not be a level that you can only get to and maintain by starvation.

I learned several years ago to find the flawlessness in my own body at different levels of development. What was essential was maintaining high levels of satisfaction in those two key areas—health and self-esteem.

A few years ago, for example, I had to learn to accept—even admire—a different kind of look for myself. For two years I scaled back my training from a competitive to a general-fitness level, and my body weight dropped dramatically. At this time my goal was to create a "normal" but athletic body that did not look overdone by weight training. I proceeded to systematically lose around fifty pounds and, of course, a great deal of that was muscle.

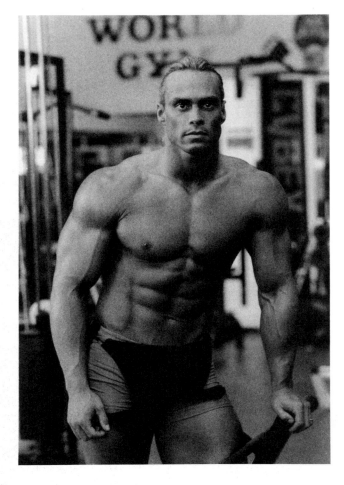

Rod Jackson's body epitomizes the athletic but noncompetitive physique possible on a Flawless program.

Also, since my workout volume was dramatically reduced, my body fat (on a day-to-day basis) increased slightly. But, I was happy with my body because I was very fit and it fulfilled my goals.

Over the next ten weeks, I want you to work toward the body that you will be happy with. It does not matter if at this moment you are overweight, underweight, experienced, or inexperienced; I want you to aim for change.

Now, I make no claim that I can take you from a novice to a Mr. America body in the next ten weeks. What I do promise you is this: If you follow the exercise and nutrition routines that I've presented here, you will see dramatic change.

All I need from you—no: All you need from yourself is a commitment to invest in your future.

Let this book act as your guide (your map and compass, so to speak). Let us hope it will be a very motivating guide. It is my wish that it will motivate you to act today. Tomorrow will always be tomorrow no matter what day it is. If you wait, you will have lost another day. You need to adopt the philosophy that gets me through those times when I feel like doing something later.

Just do it now!

So set a goal for yourself for the next ten weeks. Make your goal vivid and personal. The key to this ten-week goal is following the physical, nutritional and motivational program you select in this book as closely as possible.

The structure of the training chapters will enable you to follow your goal one day at a time.

What I'd like for you to do now is answer the following five questions with complete honesty. Choose the one answer that most applies to you. If you can't decide between two answers, choose the response that popped into your head first. That's the one that your uncluttered mind will be telling you is the right one. Please also understand that this is not a pass-or-fail test; higher or lower numbers do not mean better or worse. It's only meant as a guide to determine at what level you should be training.

Questions to Determine Training Level

A. What is your experience in training with weights?

> 1. **0-3 months**
> 2. **3-6 months**
> 3. **6 months to 2 years**
> 4. **2-5 years**
> 5. **Over 5 years**

B. What do you hope to achieve from your workouts?

  1. **Muscle tone and/or weight loss**
  2. **Muscle tone and/or weight gain**
  3. **Great beach body, but not "overdone"**
  4. **Very athletic-looking physique**
  5. **Competitive-bodybuilding physique**

C. What is the state of your health right now?

  1. **Very poor**
  2. **Poor**
  3. **Good**
  4. **Very Good**
  5. **Excellent**

D. How would you describe your body right now?

  1. **Overweight with little muscle tone**
  2. **Underweight with little muscle tone**
  3. **Medium build, somewhat fat and some muscle tone**
  4. **Plenty of muscle, but fat level too high**
  5. **Athletic with good fat-to-muscle ratio**

E. How does your body respond to exercise?

  1. **Have very little or no experience**
  2. **Slowly, with very few visual results**
  3. **Hard-gainer, but some response**
  4. **Respond to systematic routines and diets**
  5. **Lift only bricks and have 18" arms**

Now go back over your questions and add up the total points by using the number of the response on each question. For example, if you answered question A with response #1, you would get 1 point. This scale will help you determine which training section of the book you should use.

Scoring

5-12 Apprentice (beginner)
13-20 Journeyman (intermediate)
21-25 Master (advanced)

There is one exception to this self-rating, however. If you're an absolute beginner in weight training, even though your score may be out of the apprentice range, start in that section anyway. There are skills in this section that are essential for you to learn.

Before you get into your program I'd like to discuss how you should use this book to achieve the highest level of success possible. Pull out our imaginations again. Reach down inside for that childlike sense of wonder and adventure that many of us close off on our way to becoming adults tangling with the real world. This next ten-week period should be an adventure for you. Better yet, it should be like *preparing* for an adventure. You should feel as if you're ten years old and waiting for your birthday and Christmas, rolled into one spectacular occasion.

Above all, you shouldn't turn the next ten weeks into drudgery. Will you have ups and downs during the next seventy days? Of course. Some days your motivation will soar and others it will seem to drag. To that, I say, "Keep your eye on the prize." The prize is your flawless body. Along with that reward come side benefits such as self-discipline and enhanced self-esteem. Don't fear the success, crave it. Know that you will succeed and do your best. You deserve it.

I've structured this book so that there's a separate section for apprentice trainers and another for journeymen and masters. Each of these two sections is divided into one chapter for each week of the ten-week programs. I chose ten weeks as the training period because it's long enough to see real changes and short enough to sustain consistent motivation. Each chapter will contain your workouts for one week, along with tips that will be useful to your progress. At the end of the book is an Appendix that includes a section on nutrition. Read over each of the sections carefully to determine the proper nutrition program for your goals. Each serves a special purpose. Integrate the meal plan that you feel is right for you with your physical and mental exercises. Each program is set up as a whole and uniform system and should be followed as much "to the letter" as possible. Following the training advice but not following the nutrition advice will *not* accomplish your goal.

The last thing I want you to do before moving on is to write a contract with yourself for this ten-week commitment. Don't go any further until you've done this. Its purpose is to make you take responsibility for your investment. If you just say "I'll do it," you can easily change your mind. No gentleman's agreement on this, and you can't shake your own hand to seal the deal. I want it in writing and I want you to read it at least twice a day (three times on days when your motivation is lagging). So write it out, sign it and put it where you'll see it daily—on the refrigerator, in a journal recording your training results, in your briefcase; you decide. You can be elaborate in getting into goal details or you can keep it simple.

At a minimum the contract should include your name, what you're committing to, a promise to follow through and your signature. It's also a good idea to include the date that you'll begin your program and the date you'll finish. You might also consider your own personality for a minute. Are you likely to be more or less motivated by having someone share in your goal? Does the idea of having someone witness your contract make you think that you'll have another person breathing down your neck or nagging you about your goal? Do you shut down when this happens? If you do, then it's probably best to keep your contract to yourself. If having someone witnessing your contract for you—as well as asking if you're fulfilling your goals—motivates you, then have him or her sign it. It could be your spouse, girlfriend, boyfriend, training partner or anyone else you feel comfortable sharing your goal with.

Are you ready to invest in your future? I thought so!

Let's get started.

How the Muscles Work

PART ONE: MUSCLE MOVEMENT

One of the most difficult tasks in writing a book such as this is having to use words to explain sections that might be more effectively demonstrated in person. One comment that I hear from absolute beginners is how confusing it can be to translate written exercise instructions into accurate performance. This is especially true when the person doesn't really know the difference between, say, a tricep and a lat. (There's certainly nothing wrong with that, by the way. There are many people who *do* know the difference who have difficulty with exercise performance. This book is here, in part, to explain these differences.) In this section I will attempt to give simple and precise explanations of how each different body part works. I'll also include examples of exercises that best demonstrate the muscle function described. And I've worked up some rough illustrations of the torso, front and back, so that you'll know where the various muscles are in relation to each other.

I can't even begin to count the number of times I've watched as apprentice exercisers do very strange things to themselves in the gym because no one has ever told them that it's vital to isolate and feel the body part that is being worked. Just throwing the weight from point A to point B isn't enough.

I was doing a seminar at a gym recently and a very enthusiastic woman asked what I would recommend to the beginner. I said, "You should learn to perfect the exercises and feel the muscle being worked."

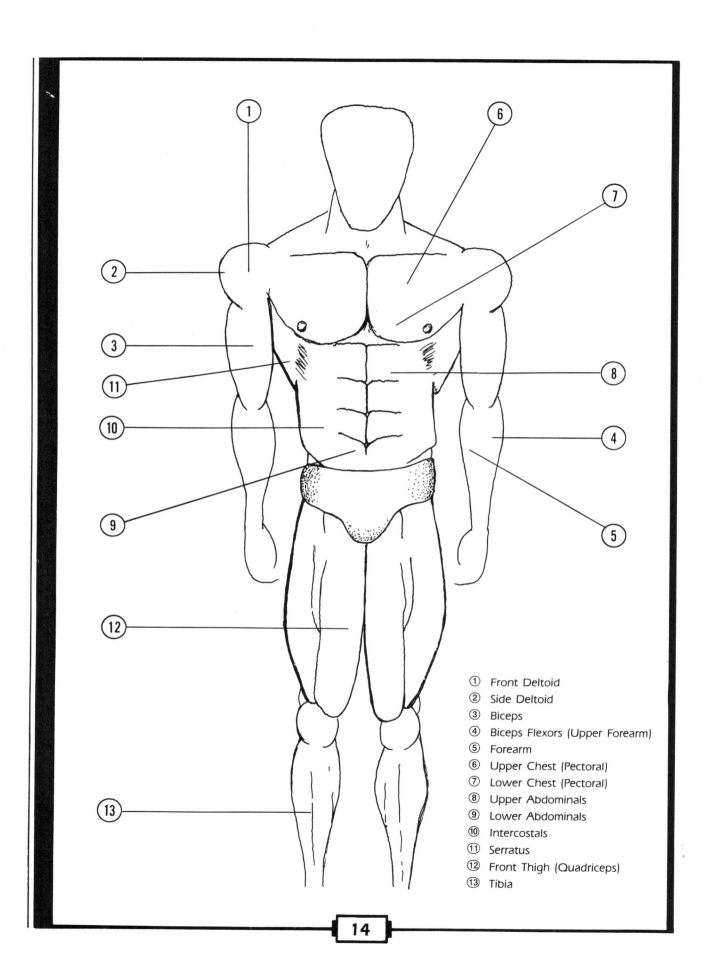

① Front Deltoid
② Side Deltoid
③ Biceps
④ Biceps Flexors (Upper Forearm)
⑤ Forearm
⑥ Upper Chest (Pectoral)
⑦ Lower Chest (Pectoral)
⑧ Upper Abdominals
⑨ Lower Abdominals
⑩ Intercostals
⑪ Serratus
⑫ Front Thigh (Quadriceps)
⑬ Tibia

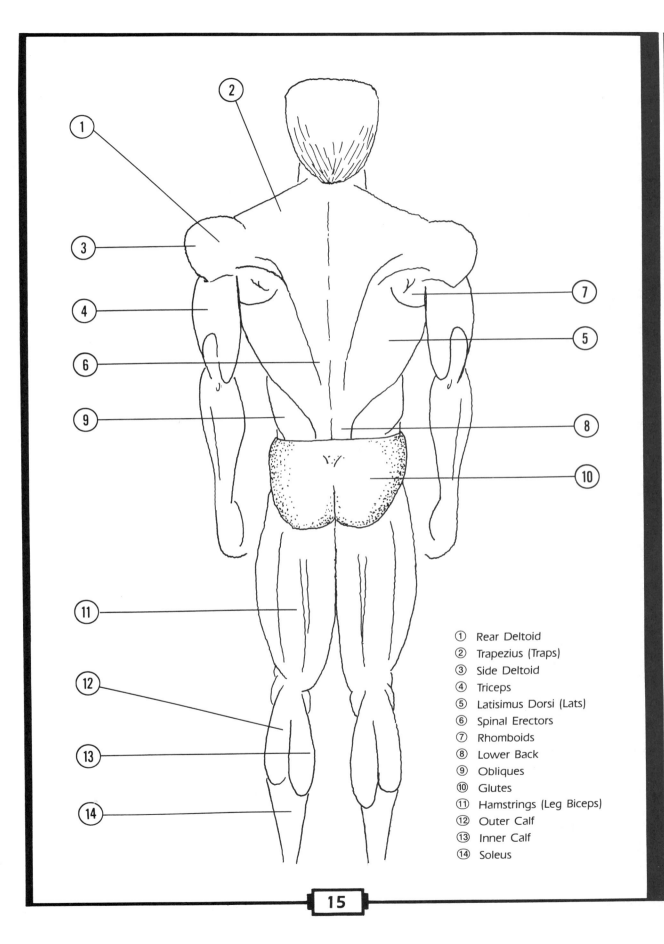

① Rear Deltoid
② Trapezius (Traps)
③ Side Deltoid
④ Triceps
⑤ Latisimus Dorsi (Lats)
⑥ Spinal Erectors
⑦ Rhomboids
⑧ Lower Back
⑨ Obliques
⑩ Glutes
⑪ Hamstrings (Leg Biceps)
⑫ Outer Calf
⑬ Inner Calf
⑭ Soleus

15

"Really?" she said, very surprised.

"Didn't anyone ever tell you that?" I asked.

"No."

You might say that exercise perfection is an obsession of mine. My motto is, "You've got to feel the muscle work to make the body respond."

Some people spend years training before realizing that they must do more than simply move the weights up and down. If you've ever played golf or tennis, you know there is a certain groove a perfect swing falls into. It's the natural path that leads to the perfect shot; it just feels right. With experience you'll know when you're performing the exercises perfectly.

I'm confused when someone asks if it's really all that important to perform the exercises perfectly. To me, it's the first step that must be made before real progress can be expected. I've overheard some very experienced pro athletes criticize my strong emphasis on perfect form. What I don't think they understand is that their bodies may be *naturally* gifted to grow, no matter what they do in the gym. That's why the best athletes don't always make the best teachers. They know what works for their own body, not what would work best for someone else.

I like to approach training from the perspective of the hard-gainer—the person who finds it difficult to reap the benefits of exercise. If I teach methods that will help the hard-gainer improve, then certainly the genetically gifted will thrive as well.

How does this perfection business apply to you and your ten-week program? Basically, it works like this. You can either waste years of your valuable time just going through the motions in the gym and get...well, basically nowhere, or you can learn right from the first day how to develop the feel in the muscle so that your time is spent productively. So spend the next seventy days spinning your wheels, or use them to create results. The choice is yours. I know which one I'd choose.

How *do* the muscles function, and how will you know if you are getting the feel of each one? You must begin at the most basic level. Each repetition of an exercise is made up of the stretched position and the contracted position. For example, the stretched position on a flat bench-press movement is when the arms are lowered and the bar is touching the chest. The contracted position is when the arms are fully extended with the bar up over the chest and the pectoral muscles flexed. The action that takes place during and between these two points is what separates a sloppy repetition from a perfect one. On almost every exercise, the weight should be lowered and raised under absolute control. This does not necessarily mean slow motion (although I recommend to people who have a tendency to do reps too fast to think in terms of "molasses on a winter day" to slow down the movement). It means fighting against the muscles being worked when moving the weight to the stretched point and using the muscles being worked to "flex" the weight into the contraction position.

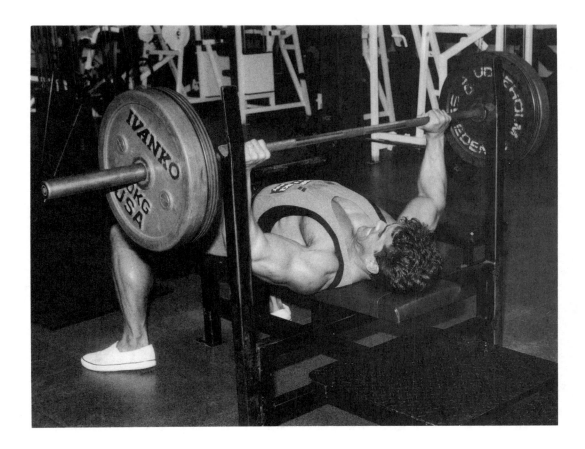

When lowering the bar on a bench press, you would fight against the weight load with your chest muscles instead of just letting the bar drop down. When you're pushing the bar away from your chest, you would begin by flexing (or contracting) the chest muscles while in the stretched position (the bar is on the chest and the pecs are fully stretched), then squeeze the chest muscles while pushing the bar back into the top of the movement. At the top of the movement you would not begin to lower the weight again until you had found a tremendous contraction in the chest muscle.

These are difficult concepts for some people to understand, and even harder for most to practice. It's much easier to just move the weights around without focusing on the muscles. However, as I said before, you'll get a small fraction of the full benefit that *feeling* the reps will give you.

There's also a difference between the way a power lifter (someone who is only concerned with moving a certain weight from point A to point B) does a bench press and the method I just described, which will work best for someone trying to improve his or her physical appearance. The competitive power lifter is primarily concerned with the ability to lift the weight, not with how the pec muscles will develop as a result of the exercise. You'll be trying to sculpt your body with the weight, so control and contraction are essential.

There is an entirely separate reason to learn exercise perfection that we haven't discussed yet: It will be very difficult to injure yourself if you're performing the exercises just right. Weight-training injuries usually come from either sloppy form or overuse of the joint, tendon, muscle and/or bone structure.

The first type of injury is what I'll call a ballistic injury—for example, throwing your back out when you bend over to pick something up the wrong way or waking up with a kink in your neck from sleeping in a funny position. The second type occurs due to inadequate recovery from your workouts, and can easily be compounded by a ballistic injury.

Let's talk now about the individual body parts and the best way you can go about learning how to make them work over the next ten weeks and beyond.

HOW THE CHEST WORKS

On their most basic level, the chest muscles perform two main functions. The first involves the actions of pushing the body away from something—picture a push-up, for example. With a push-up you are pushing your body away from the floor. The chest muscles are the primary moving force. The stretch point would be when your chest touches the floor. The contraction position is when your arms are extended fully and the chest is flexed. Now, on almost every exercise you will be working primary and secondary muscles. With chest-pressing movements (any action where you're pushing something away from the body), the primary muscle is the chest, but there are also two joint movements involved—that of the elbow joint and the shoulder joint. Therefore, support muscles for these joints are called into play and become secondary muscles that are being worked. In this case the secondary muscles being worked would be the triceps and the front deltoids (the muscles surrounding the shoulder joint). The focus when doing a chest-press movement should be on the chest, but these secondary muscles will inevitably get some work also.

Chest-press movements can be done at a variety of angles, from incline to flat to decline. Incline movements work with upper chest from the clavicles to mid-chest. Flat movements affect the mid to lower chest, and decline exercises mostly work the lower chest.

The second main function of the chest involves bringing the arms across in front of the body. Picture standing with your arms extended out to the sides, parallel to the ground. Now move your arms forward until your hands come together in front of your chest. Push your hands together hard. Do you feel the contraction in the chest muscles? This is the action of the chest that is involved in performing a dumbbell-flye movement.

When doing exercises of this type it's important to keep your elbows slightly bent. If you were to keep your elbows locked straight you would put too much stress on the elbow joint and would probably eventually injure the area. Because these movements don't involve a full stretch at the elbow joint, the triceps are not involved the way they are on a pressing exercise. So, the main secondary muscles worked are the front deltoids.

It is essential, by the way, when doing either pressing or flye exercises, to keep your shoulders in their natural position. Many people have a tendency to push their shoulders forward when doing a chest movement. This will prevent the chest from being fully isolated and flexed. You can correct and check this shoulder positioning with a simple practice technique. Extend your arms in front of the body; put your hands together and press inward until you isolate the contraction in your chest. Extend your hands forward until your shoulders push forward also. Now bring your shoulders back into their natural position (not pushed forward or backward and not shrugged up). That is where they should be during the contraction point of chest exercises. Anytime you feel you aren't "finding" your chest during a workout, stop and use this practice technique to get back in touch with the right feeling.

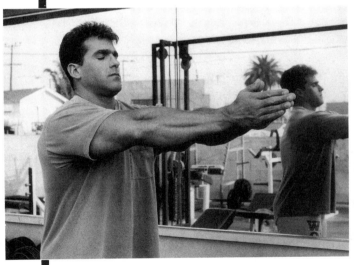

Pushing the shoulders forward *prevents* proper isolation on a chest-pressing movement.

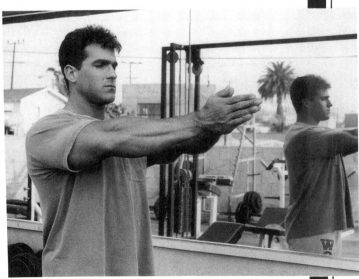

Try to keep the shoulders back in their natural position.

HOW THE BACK WORKS

The area referred to as the back covers a lot of territory on your body. Its muscles stretch from the base of the neck to the top of the butt and go from shoulder to shoulder. Most people find the back muscles very hard to get the feel of when training. I partially attribute this to the inability to see the back while working out. You don't have the visual contact you have when you're training the chest, for example, and can see it working in the gym mirror. The importance of monitoring muscle movement is one of the reasons there are so many mirrors in most gyms. They are not just there, as a critic might claim, for narcissistic reasons. Rather, they allow trainers to correct exercise form and further enhance the physical contractions with visual feedback. It is rather like a biofeedback loop. The more you see, the more you feel—the greater the result.

It can be helpful to use mental-image techniques to create a mirror in your mind and watch your back work. Of course, the more you know about how the back functions in various exercises, the better you'll be at creating this imaginary mirror.

Before describing the back's three basic functions, let's talk about isolating the back muscles. Isolation, when used in bodybuilding language, means to separate the primary muscle from the secondary muscles and the rest of the body as much as possible. On nearly every back exercise, your arms will provide the link that will attach you to the weights. Many people find it difficult to take their arms out of the action and put the isolation on the back. You should think of your arms merely as hooks that attach to the weight. Think of this system as being similar to a construction crane. The crane's engine represents your back muscles. The cable and hook represent your arms and hands, and the object attached to the hook represents the weight being lifted. In this situation, it is the crane's engine that does all of the work. The cable and hook provide the crane with the link and ability to move a certain amount of weight from point A to point B. And, although stress is placed on the cable and hook, they are very secondarily involved in the object's movement. They are important parts of the system, yes, but only in the sense of giving the engine the ability to perform its task.

The first of the three basic exercise functions of the back is the pull-down/pull-up motion. This involves setting the upper body in an upright position and either pulling the body up toward a bar (as in a pull-up) or pulling a bar (attached to a cable, pulley and weight system) down toward the body (a pull-down movement).

On a pull-up, the stretch position is when the body is hanging with the arms fully extended. In this position your shoulders will seem to be dislocated.

They aren't really, of course; they're just stretched upward toward the ears. The body's hanging creates a stretch in the primary muscles for this exercise, the lats.

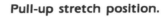

Pull-up stretch position.

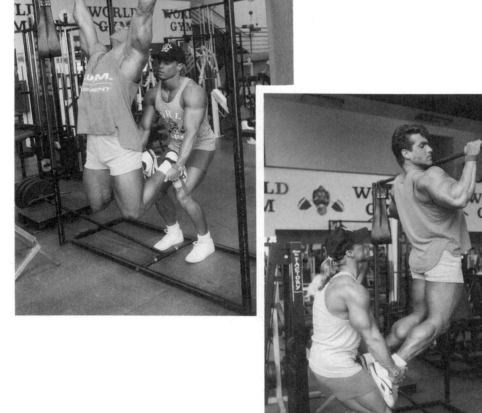

Pull-up contraction position.

The contraction position is when the body is pulled up to the bar and all of the back muscles are flexed. The complicated part is getting from the stretch to the contraction while isolating the back as much as possible.

A pull-up or pull-down movement consists of four steps:

1. Stretch point—The arms are fully extended, the lat muscles are stretched and the shoulders are up toward the ears.

2. Pushing the shoulders down—On a pull-up this will involve pulling the body upward, with arms still fully extended, by pulling the shoulders down into their natural position. The shoulder joints will go from their "dislocated" stretched position down into their natural place. To demonstrate this movement, raise one extended arm straight up in the air. Now extend your arm farther, as if grabbing for an object six inches above your fingertips. Keep your body stationary and just reach up with your arm. You'll see that your shoulder joint travels up with the arm. Now pull your shoulder joint back down to where it also began. It's like a three- or four-inch shrug with the shoulder. When you pull your shoulder joints into place on a pull-up, you are putting the lat muscles into their most efficient position for contraction.

3. Pulling upward—With the shoulder joint pulled down in position, you will pull yourself up toward the bar. As you are pulling the body up imagine that you are pulling the bar down toward your body. At the same time imagine that you are going to touch your elbows to your sides when you get to the top. Now, of course, since you're holding on to a bar or handle, this will be impossible. But, if you try to touch your elbows to your sides at the top, all the back muscles will contract. Make sure to find this contraction before moving on to the next step.

4. Returning to the stretch—Once the contraction happens, fight against your body weight and lower yourself back to the hanging stretched position.

These four steps represent one repetition. With practice each of the four steps will flow smoothly into one another. In general, pull-down or pull-up exercises affect the width of the back and can be done with a wide, medium or narrow hand spacing. On medium- and wide-grip movements, the bar can be pulled down to the front or behind the neck. Any change in grip space or front/rear style has a slightly different effect on the area of muscle emphasized. I'll go over these differences in specific exercise descriptions in later chapters.

The second back function is pulling objects toward the body with the arms extended in front of the torso. This action is best represented by rowing movements; in fact, the action very much physically resembles rowing a boat.

The muscle function is to shrug the shoulder blades together in the middle of the back. Picture trying to squeeze an orange between your shoulder blades. The stretch position on a rowing movement is arms extended forward, with the shoulders "dislocated" once again so that the back muscles are fully extended.

In learning the rowing function, you'll be following the same steps that I described in the pull-up section. One major difference comes in step 3, though. Instead of trying to touch your elbows to your sides, as in a pull-up, you want to pull your elbows back as far as possible at the contraction point. It's as if you're trying to touch your elbows together behind your back. Of course, you can't physically do this, but it gives you a mental image of how to contract the muscles.

The main difference between pull-ups and rows is the angle of the arm extension. The arms are extended overhead for pull-ups and in front of the body for rows. The action of shrugging the shoulder blades is what makes rowing movements unique. This movement works mainly to increase the thickness of the back structure. Rowing movements can be done from a number of different angles and with different equipment. The most basic movements are barbell rows and seated pulley rows.

The third basic exercise group can best be called rotation exercises. Here, the action focuses on the rotation of the shoulder joint. The back muscles are flexed by rotating the arms (at the shoulder joint) in an arc along the sides of the body. The best exercise to show this action is a straight-arm pull-in. The term "straight-arm" is not really an accurate description. Actually your arms should be slightly bent and locked in that position throughout the range of motion. This exercise is performed with a high-pulley, weight-stack machine (lat pull-down or tricep push-down station) and medium-length bar, and can be done standing or kneeling. The stretched position would be with your arms (in that bent and locked position) extended in front and your hands just above the top of your head, so that the back muscles are stretching. Your shoulders should be down in a natural position, as opposed to shrugged upward. Now think in terms of your hands following a semicircular arc down and back until the bar touches the front of your thighs. On this exercise you must have your back arched (stick your butt out) and your chest lifted to create a flex.

Try this flex now without a weight. Stand upright, and arch your back by sticking your butt out and lifting your chest. Now press the palms of your hands against the front of your thighs and push your elbows back as if trying to touch them to the wall behind you. You should feel your back flexing. Your elbows should not be pointing out to the sides. They should be parallel to each other throughout the movement, as if your arms are on a roller-coaster track and your elbows are attached to that track through the arc of the exercise.

In each of these three basic functions, your back was the primary area being worked. The secondary muscles activated in pull-up and rowing exercises are the biceps and the rear deltoid. They are both activated in a similar way to the triceps and front deltoids on chest exercises. This is because of the two-jointed nature of these exercises involving the elbow and shoulder joints. On rotation exercises, only the rear deltoid has a secondary effect. The biceps are not really involved, since there is no pulling toward the body.

Your back muscles can be very difficult to flex in the beginning, but like all skills the feeling can be perfected with time, repetition and attention to detail. You'll discover that once you learn how to feel a muscle group work, it will be impossible to do a movement incorrectly again without feeling like you're cheating yourself.

HOW THE BICEPS WORK

The primary biceps function is to assist the elbow in bending and bringing the hand and forearm toward the body. The secondary function is to rotate the hand and forearm from a palm-up to a palm-down position, and vice versa. This secondary action of rotating the wrist is called supination. The supination of your hand will determine what part of the biceps will be worked and how intense the direct biceps contraction will be. The farther your hand is turned outward at the top of a biceps exercise, the greater the direct flex will be. If your palm is facing in during the exercise, you'll be working more outer biceps and the top of your forearm.

Supination is a technique used to stretch the biceps at the bottom of a curling movement by turning the palms inward toward the body in the stretch position. Of course, you can only supinate your wrist when working each arm independently of the other, as in a dumbbell or single-arm cable curl. That's why most intermediate and advanced routines are composed of a mixture of dumbbell and barbell movements.

All this talk about supination means nothing without further exploring the primary biceps function. With very few exceptions, the primary biceps exercises fall into the category of curls. In fact, even the exceptions (under-handed pull-ups, for example) are a sort of cockeyed curl, in that the physiological function very nearly duplicates what you would do to flex your biceps while performing a barbell curl.

On curls, the stretched position is when the arm is fully extended and an essentially straight line runs from the shoulder joint, through the elbow and down to the wrist. In this stretched position the bicep is extended to its fullest length, attaching at the top just under the front deltoid and at the bottom just above the inside of the elbow joint. The contraction point will be where the biceps is shortened and flexed.

The biceps gives us one of the clearest examples of how contraction (the shortening of the muscle) actually lifts the weight. Stick your arm out straight in front. Now turn your palm in and bend your elbow so that you touch your hand to the shoulder opposite the arm extended (Position A). Watch your biceps muscles as you do this. Notice how it goes from being long and stretched when your arm is extended to being short and bunched-up when touching the shoulder. Now do this same movement but press against the palm with the other hand to create enough tension so you can feel the biceps work (Position B). That is the feeling you want to get during curling exercises.

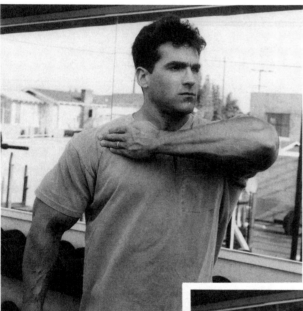

Position A.

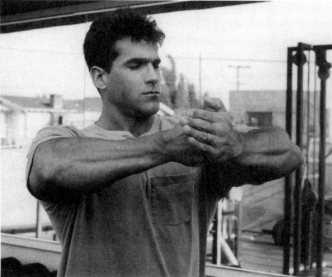

Position B.

The secondary muscles worked on curls are the forearms and the front deltoid. As you might have noticed, some part of the deltoid is a secondary muscle on all upper-body movements that involve holding the weights (or a bar or handle attached to the weights in your hands). This is one reason why shoulder injuries are so prevalent in weight training. These "overuse injuries" can be avoided through strict exercise style and by allowing adequate recuperation between workouts.

When working your biceps it's important to keep your shoulders out of the movement as much as possible. It's easy to get the front deltoid overly involved if you're not focused on isolating the biceps muscles.

HOW THE TRICEPS WORK

Your triceps muscles have two basic functions; the first we'll call "pressing" and the second "extending." I've already described how triceps are the secondary muscle used on chest-pressing movements. When performing triceps-pressing exercises, both the chest and the front deltoid becomes secondary to the flex you're trying to find in your triceps.

As it turns out, the pressing movements for triceps are nearly identical to chest-press exercises. They usually differ in hand spacing, elbow placement and body position. They also differ in where you place your mental concentration during the execution.

A closer-grip bench press is an example of a triceps-press movement. Your hands would be placed much closer together on the bar than in a regular bench press, but the stretch position would still be the same. In the case of close-grip bench presses, the arms follow a different path between stretch and contraction. In the chest-press movement the upper arms are positioned with the elbows pointing straight out. In the correct position you can draw a straight line from one elbow to the other and the line will travel through both shoulder joints as well. It will seem as if you're pulling your elbows back in order to get this position. In close-grip bench-press movement, though, the elbows are brought closer together, so that when the bar is touching the chest in the stretch position, the forearms should almost be touching the sides of the waist.

The contraction position has the arms extended up over the chest, with the flex concentrated on the back of the upper arm. Only after finding the contraction should you lower the bar back to your chest, using the triceps' strength to resist the weight.

Many people have a difficult time finding the triceps contraction on this exercise. If your elbows are locked when your arms are fully extended, you may be creating a crutchlike structure for the weight to rest on, without fully flexing the triceps. In such a case, the weight will rest on this straight-line bone structure and the muscle won't be effectively contracted. The solution lies in not quite locking the elbows out. Instead, go to a point about a millimeter from lockout, so that your arms are fully extended but the weight remains on the muscle structure.

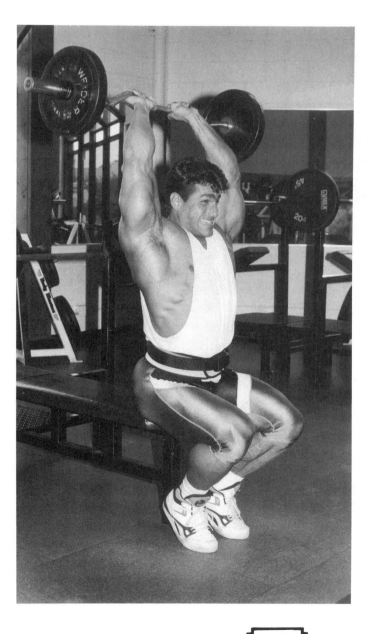

As with the close-grip bench press, the French press should be performed with elbows not quite locked out, thereby keeping the tension on the muscle.

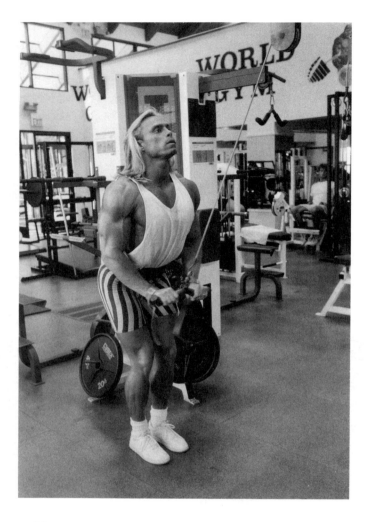

The second triceps function is best executed with extension-type movements. In the case of triceps-press movements, as exemplified by the close-grip bench press, you were using two joint actions to perform the movement. You had a bend at the elbows, and the shoulder joints moved along with the arm. Extension exercises, when done strictly, involved the joint action of the elbow only.

Whereas the biceps function was to raise the forearm toward the upper arm, your triceps' second function is to extend the forearm away from the upper arm. Biceps bend the arm; triceps straighten it. So the stretched position for extending exercises is the elbow bent and the forearm touching the biceps.

A good example of this function is a triceps push-down. Standing upright—and using a short-bar, cable high-pulley and weight system—you keep your elbows close at your side. Upper arms are to remain in place throughout the movement from stretch to contraction. Bending at the elbow, the forearm touches the biceps. The contraction would be with the bar pushed downward until the hands are in front of the thighs and the elbow is straightened. Once again, just go slightly short of a full lockout and squeeze throughout the whole movement. The triceps should be flexed as much as possible. So when raising the bar back up to the stretch position, fight against the weight. When starting to push the bar down toward contraction, begin by contracting the triceps as hard as possible in the stretch position and then flex the weight down.

Extension movements have only the front deltoid as a minor secondary muscle. The forearms are also activated by grabbing the bar, but this is true on any exercise when you use your hands to grab the weight.

HOW THE SHOULDERS WORK

As you have seen in the discussion of the preceding four body parts, shoulders play an integral role in almost all upper-body exercises. The ball-and-socket joint allows the deltoid to assist every time you reach out to grab something, scratch your head, pet your dog or pour a cup of tea. The functions of the deltoid muscle are to raise the arms laterally, rotate the arms and push objects away from the body.

The lateral movement can be done in basically any direction—straight in front, to the side or to the rear. To demonstrate this, hang your arms by your side, palms facing in. Now raise your arms slowly and under muscular control, with your palms facing the floor, until your elbows are on the same level as your shoulder joints. The same arm motion done holding weights can be done to affect the front, side and rear deltoid. For rear-deltoid movements, the upper body is usually bent forward at the waist, and the lateral movement is still moving the arms from their hanging position up till the elbows are as high as—and lined up with—the shoulder joint.

The stretch position on laterals is when the arms are hanging down, and the contraction point is when the arms are raised. In all lateral movements, it's essential to slightly bend at the elbows to avoid stress injury to the area. Also, since one of the deltoid functions involves rotating the arms, you'll want to slightly tip the dumbbell forward, like you're pouring water out of a bottle, at the contraction point of the movement. This will greatly intensify the muscle contraction.

It can be very hard to hold the contractions on lateral movements, so it's essential to use a weight that allows you to do the movements slowly and under complete control. Fight the weight down when lowering and squeeze the weight up to the top.

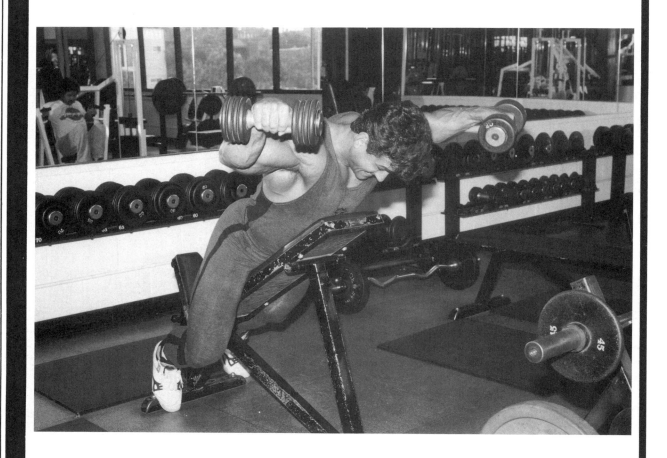

The next function involves pushing objects away from the body. You've already seen how this function is accomplished in connection with the other body parts. This pushing-away motion is why the front deltoids are so activated on chest and triceps presses. However, in order to turn the deltoid into the primary working muscle, you'll need to press in a different direction. Shoulder presses will have you moving the weight straight overhead. I'll use dumbbell presses as the exercise example here. The stretch position on this exercise would be when the arms are bent at the elbow so that the hands and dumbbells are on the same level as the deltoid. In this position, the deltoid muscles are fully expanded and stretched. The delts are also in position to push those dumbbells back overhead. Think of this position as being like a slingshot with the rubber band pulled all the way back poised to release its energy. In fact, a good visualization technique for pressing movements of all kinds is to imagine that as the weight is lowering, the muscle is building up energy to drive it right back up to the top—sort of like a spring being compressed and then released.

Start by flexing the deltoid muscles in the stretched position and squeeze the weight up into the contraction position.

An important factor in the proper performance of shoulder presses is upper-arm placement. You want your elbows pulled back into a similar position used for chest pressing. Remember how you should be able to draw a straight line from one elbow to the other, with that line bisecting the shoulder joints. If your elbows are forward, the movement becomes more dependent on triceps—which, by the way, are the secondary muscle on shoulder presses because of their role in straightening the arm.

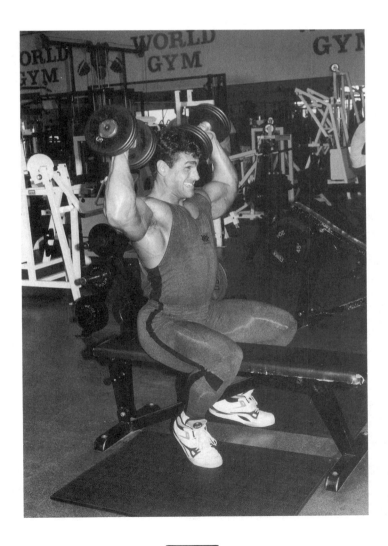

The deltoid contraction occurs when the weight is overhead and the arms are fully extended. Once again I want you to do just a hair short of full lockout so that you don't rest the weight on the bone-structure "crutch" that is created. This way the tension stays on the deltoid muscle.

Throughout the movement, make sure that your shoulder joints are down in their natural position instead of shrugged up to your ears. When you get to the top of the movement, rotate your arms just slightly at the shoulders, as if trying to turn your thumbs to face out away from the body. Your elbows will go back about half an inch. This very slight movement will feel like the top of a lateral raise and will increase the deltoid flex intensity. Before lowering the weights, move your arms back into their original position.

HOW THE FRONT THIGHS WORK

There is a remarkable similarity between the muscles of your upper and lower limbs. The knee- and elbow-joint movements are similar. The hip and shoulder joints are both ball-and-socket structures. So it should be no surprise that your front thigh's place in the leg structure resembles your triceps' place on its own, or that the basic functions of the two muscle groups are nearly identical. The two functions of your front thigh revolve around one concept: to straighten the leg from a bent-knee position. Just like with triceps, the two functions are pressing and extending. The difference between the two actions are that pressing involves two joint actions (knee and hip) and extending only one (knee).

Once again the pressing involves pushing away from the body or pushing the body away from something. The prime example of pushing the body away from something is a squat. You're pushing your body away from the floor by standing up from a squatting position. A leg press would be an example of pushing something away from the body.

The stretch position on a leg press occurs when the legs are lowered so that they're touching the chest. The front thigh muscles are fully stretched because of the bend in the knees.

The secondary muscles worked on leg-pressing movements are the gluteus muscles, lower back and leg biceps. The glutes, in fact, operate in a way that is similar to the action of the deltoid in an upper-body movement. When the weight is lowered into the stretch, the glutes are pulled tight because of the joints bending and will assist the front thigh in pushing the weight to the contraction position.

The contraction position is with the knee straightened. The difficult part for many people is finding a solid flex in the front thigh at the top of a leg-pressing movement. You'll want to avoid the bone-structure "crutch" dilemma described in the triceps section by once again pushing until you're a millimeter short of fully locking out the knees.

So that you'll understand how to flex the front thigh on a press movement, let's talk for a moment about an extension movement. The primary exercise for the job is a description of itself—a leg extension.

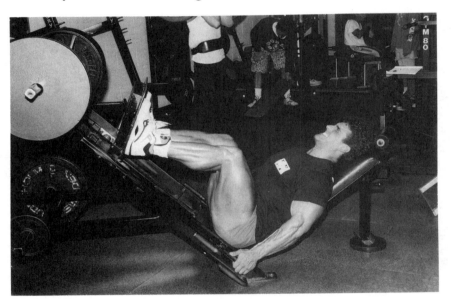

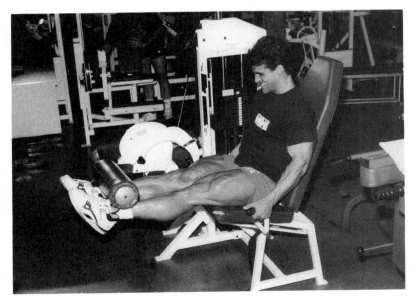

Going for full contraction on leg extensions.

The contraction point on a leg extension happens when the knee is straightened and a straight line runs from the ankle to the hip. It's the last few inches of this movement that really flex the front thigh, though. That's because the muscle is coming from such a stretched state and really bunching up for a contraction.

It's usually easier for people to find a front-thigh flex on leg extensions than on presses. So when you're doing your pressing exercises, I want you to mentally transfer the feeling that you get on the extension to the contraction of the press. In that last four or five inches before you get to the top of a leg press, imagine that you're straightening your knees into the last few inches of a leg extension.

Pressing movements can be done from a variety of different angles and foot positions. Whenever you change your foot position, always make sure that your kneecaps are pointing in the same direction as your toes. This prevents any twisting of the knee-joint structure, maintains alignment and prevents injury.

We've talked already about the flex position for extensions. Let's now discuss the stretch.

The stretch happens when the knee is bent and the front thigh is pulled taut; sitting on a leg-extension machine, this would mean when your feet are pointing toward the floor. You make the exercise more effective when you keep a solid tension going in the front thigh throughout the range of motion. That stretch position should always be like a compressed spring just waiting to be unleashed.

HOW THE HAMSTRINGS WORK

If front thighs are the triceps of the leg structure, then hamstrings are the biceps. That's why they're also called leg biceps. They, like the arm biceps, are perfect examples of how the shortening and lengthening of the muscle raises and lowers the weight.

The leg-biceps function is to bend the knee and bring the heels toward the butt. Because the glute muscles are so strong, they can interfere with the hamstring contraction if the exercises are not done correctly.

There are two main ways that hamstrings are worked. The first involves curling movements, such as the lying leg curl. The second is the type of stretching movement accomplished with stiff-leg deadlifts. The stretch position for hamstrings is the same as the contraction position for front thighs. In fact, it's that way for all opposing muscle groups in the body. The opposing muscles are: biceps and triceps; front thighs and hamstrings; abdominals and lower back (and, to a lesser extent, chest and back); and front and rear deltoid.

It is vital to develop equivalent strength on both sides of the opposition. This is not just for visual balance, but will also prevent injuries that occur when opposing muscle imbalances are present. When your knees are completely straightened, the hamstrings are pulled taut. On a lying leg curl, this would be with your legs extended. It's important to flex the hamstrings in this position also. Remember that it's the flexing and shortening of the muscle that exerts the force to raise the weight and that it is the muscle's

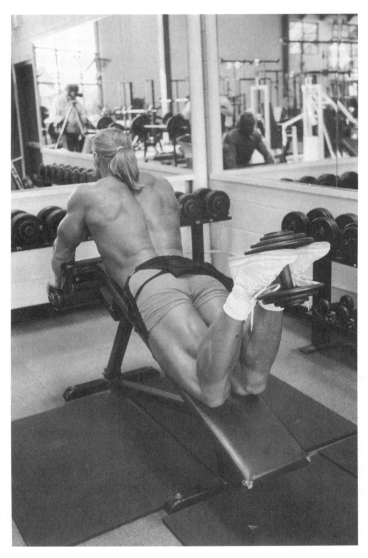

Leg curls performed with a dumbbell are an alternative for those training at home.

resistance against the weight that makes the body part grow stronger and more developed.

The contraction on leg curls comes when the leg biceps is shortened, with the knees bent and the calves pulled up toward the hamstring. The most important thing is to minimize the glute muscle's secondary influence by pushing your hips down toward the bench at the contraction point. If your butt is sticking up in the air, you won't be isolating hamstrings. You'll need to experiment to find where your hamstrings flex the best. For some it's when the calves are really pressed against the hamstring. For most, though, the maximum flex will come a couple of inches short of this. Feel your way through the movement and keep your hips pushed into the bench to find your best flex.

Stiff-leg deadlifts take the stretch farther than is possible, say, in a lying leg curl. Your knees must be locked as much as possible throughout. The stretch comes in bending the upper body forward, not from the waist but from the hip joint, until the bar touches the top of your feet. The lower back and glutes are the secondary muscles on this exercise. You can squeeze back up to the top on this exercise by flexing your glutes as you raise back into the stand-up position. There is no definite contraction on this exercise. The idea is to carefully push the stretch past its normal limits and to flex the hamstrings throughout the movement.

HOW THE CALVES WORK

The calf muscles have one main function: They are a major part of the system that gives mobility to the foot. The calves are the forearms of the lower limbs.

The calf muscles enable you to use your feet to walk, run and go up on your toes. In fact, it is this "going up on the toes" that forms the core of calf exercises. In the stretch position on a calf raise, the ankle is bent so that the toes are pointing up in the air. This is best accomplished by standing on a platform or block high enough to allow you to fully stretch the muscle without touching your heels to the ground. Your toes and the ball of the foot should be on the platform and your heels should hang off the back. Then, to put it simply, you go up on your toes. It is in this position that you'll find the contraction.

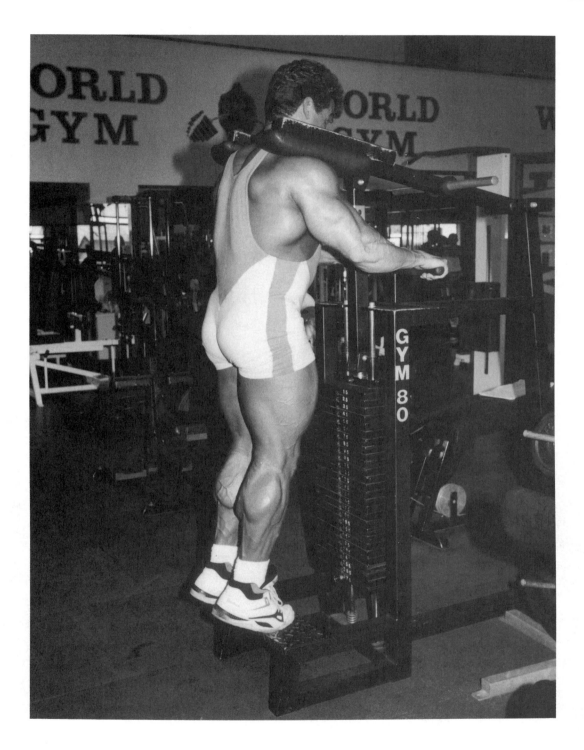

You must focus on the calf muscles, and not just the up-and-down movement, in order to flex the muscle. I've watched people spend years just raising the weights up and down before realizing that mental focus is essential to isolating any muscle being worked. Calves are no exception.

HOW THE ABDOMINALS WORK

Your abdominals can be divided into two distinct sets of muscles. The first set is made up of the plates of muscle on the front of the stomach; they're considered the abdominal muscles proper. The second set consists of the intercostal muscles on the side of your waist.

The abdominals' key function is to shorten the length between the rib cage and the pelvis. To demonstrate this action, place one finger of your left hand about three inches below your navel. With your right hand, place a finger on your sternum bone (the bottom-center of where your ribs meet) and stand up straight (Position A). Now try to shorten the distance between the two fingers. As you can see, the only way possible is by bowing your shoulders forward and curving the spine (Position B). In this way the distance is reduced and the abdominals will, with focused effort, flex.

Position A.

Position B.

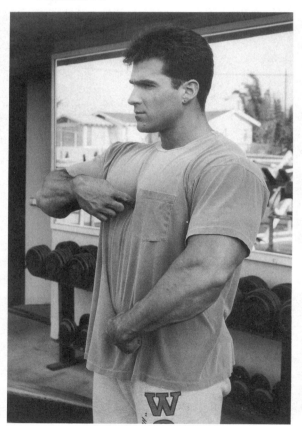

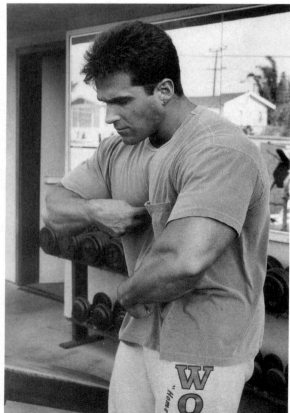

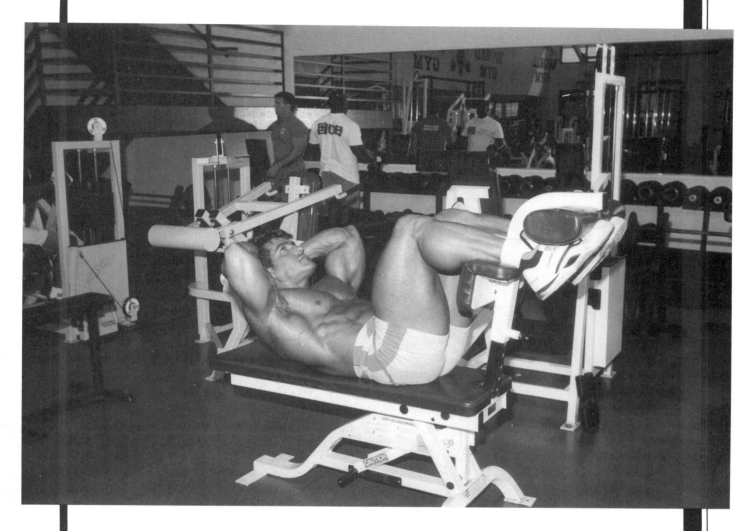

Crunch contraction position.

Within this shortening function, there are two ways to accomplish the task and to stress different sections of the abdominal muscles.

The first is a crunch-type movement. The crunch is the exercise that replaced the old-fashioned sit-up, which was not only difficult to perform correctly, but dangerous and overrated. The crunch works the top half of the abdominal wall primarily and affects the lower abdominals secondarily, and is a rather limited-range movement.

The stretch on this movement consists of lying on your back with your spine straight and your head on the ground. The contraction is simply raising your head and curling your spine until the distance between the pelvis and sternum is shortened. Throwing your body is not necessary and, in fact, can be dangerous to your lower back.

The lower abdominals are primarily worked by shortening the pelvis/sternum length as you raise and lower your legs from the hip joints. The upper abdominals play a secondary role in the leg-raise exercises. A lying leg raise best demonstrates this function.

The stretch position on a leg raise is when the legs are lowered to a position just below parallel to the ground. For this reason, it's best to do a lying leg raise with your legs extended over the end of an exercise bench.

The contraction position is when the legs are raised to an angle just above parallel to the ground. The legs will raise by a rotation at your hip joints, and your knees should be slightly bent and locked in place.

You must really focus to find the abdominal feel on leg raises. It would be easy to just move your legs up and down and totally miss your abdominals.

Crunches and leg raises can be performed from a wide variety of angles. Once you're past the beginnings of the apprentice stage, you should build routines that revolve around at least one upper and lower abdominal exercise.

The secondary abdominal function involves the intercostal muscles and represents one of the most misunderstood aspects of weight training. Intercostals rotate the waist and bend it from side to side. The problem lies in the way many people work these muscles and in the way many "experts" recommend these muscles be worked. The intercostals are best worked by doing *slight* twisting movements on crunch exercises.

The absolutely best thing you can do in the gym if you want to ruin the appearance of your body is perform weighted side bends. Any exercise where you hold a weight and bend side to side might strengthen your intercostals, but it'll also cause them to grow wider. Look, I'll keep this simple and to the point: Unless you want your waist to be as wide as your shoulders, avoid weighted side bends at all costs. Those who tell you differently don't know what they're talking about.

Please understand also that it's a myth that abdominal exercises will reduce fat on your waist. Abdominal exercises tone and build the waist muscles. Muscle and fat are two entirely different chemical compounds. One cannot "turn" into the other. Fat cannot become muscle or vice versa.

Use abdominal exercises to tone the muscle, and weight workouts, aerobics and good nutrition to reduce your body fat. The combination will make your abdominal muscles look the way you want them to.

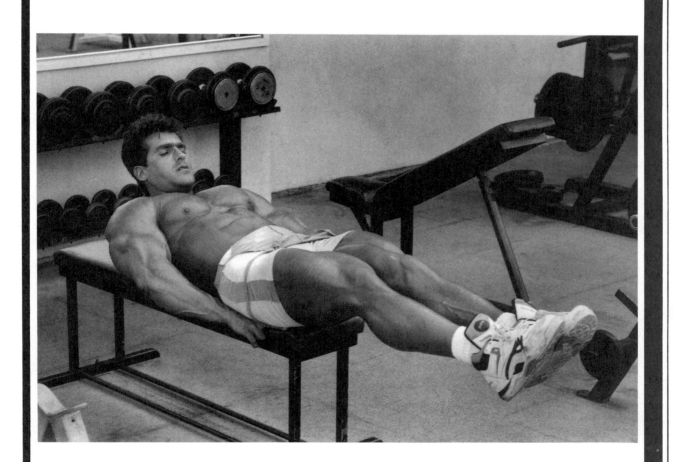

Leg-Raise stretch position.

PART TWO:
APPRENTICE EXERCISES

In this section are the performance descriptions of all the exercises you will use during the ten-week Apprentice Program. These instructions are intended to help you not only to target the primary muscle on each exercise, but also to practice perfect exercise form. The descriptions are coordinated with photos that show correct body positioning and identify necessary gym equipment.

Each description is referenced to six headings. Briefly, an explanation of those headings:

1. Primary Muscle—The body part and section of that muscle that are primarily affected by an exercise. This is the area that you should focus your mental and physical attention on as you perform your sets and repetitions.

2. Equipment—The gym equipment necessary to do the exercise.

3. Stretch—A term used in the previous chapter, the stretch position is when the muscle is at its fullest length. Usually this indicates the beginning point of an exercise.

4. Contraction—The point at which the primary muscle is flexed to its shortest dimension. The exact opposite of the stretched position.

5. Performance—A reference to the way the muscle gets from stretch to contraction and back again. Also, the special body positions that each exercise may need.

6. Variation—Any alteration of the core exercise that may, in turn, alter the area of the primary muscle that is worked. For example, if the flat bench press is the exercise being discussed, then an incline bench press would be a variation of that exercise. In this case the variation would require a different bench to be used and would work a different part of the same muscle.

The Apprentice Program consists of thirty-six different muscles rotated on a daily basis. (Of course, on no day will you be performing all thirty-six.) Eighteen of those exercises will be described in this six-step manner and represent the core exercises of your routines. The other eighteen are variations on the core exercises and will be described in the "Variations" category of the exercise performance descriptions. This, however, does not make those eighteen variations less important than the eighteen core exercises. Remember to also use Part One of "How the Muscles Work" (page 13) as a reference if you're having difficulty figuring out an exercise.

FLAT BENCH PRESSES

1. Primary Muscle—Overall chest, with emphasis on the lower half.
2. Equipment—A flat bench with uprights to support a barbell and weights.
3. Stretch—With a hand spacing approximately six to eight inches wider than shoulder width, the bar is lowered until it touches at mid to upper chest. Elbows should be kept pulled back so that they are directly under the hands.
4. Contraction—The arms are fully extended with the elbows just a millimeter short of fully locking out. Keep tension on chest muscles by flexing the chest and keeping the shoulders from pushing forward.
5. Performance—From the stretch position, begin pushing the weight away from the chest by flexing the chest muscles and extending the arms. The rib cage should be raised, but the lower back should not be arched off the bench. Keep the feet planted on the ground and the body steady as the weight is raised and lowered under control.
6. Variation—Incline bench press. Use an incline bench at a 45-degree angle with a barbell to affect the upper-chest area from the collarbones to mid-chest. Do not arch the lower back and hips off of the bench during the exercise.

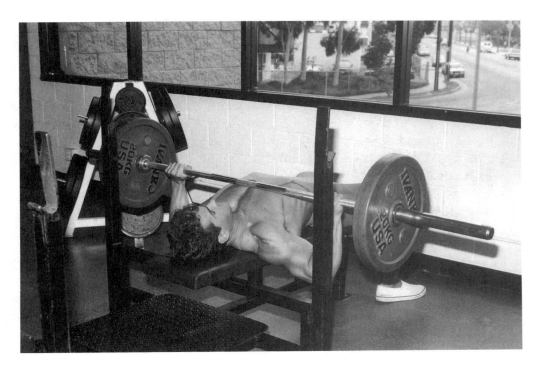

Flat Bench Press stretch position.

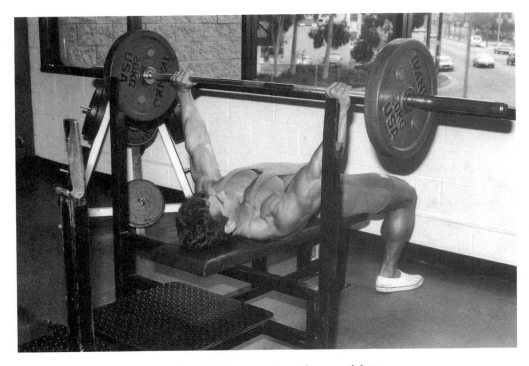

Flat Bench Press contraction position.

FLAT FLYES

1. **Primary Muscle**—Overall chest, with emphasis on lower half.
2. **Equipment**—Two dumbbells and a flat exercise bench.
3. **Stretch**—With elbows bent at a 45-degree angle, the dumbbells should be lowered out and away from the body to chest level. The elbows should be pulled back to the same vertical plane as the hands.
4. **Contraction**—The dumbbells should be touching above the chest, with the arms straightened only slightly from the 45-degree bent position. The chest should be flexed with the shoulders down and not pushed forward.
5. **Performance**—On a flye, the dumbbells follow an arc as they are moved from a side position (stretch) to a narrow position (contraction). The rib cage should be lifted without arching the lower back and there should be the feeling of bringing the arms across the body instead of pushing a weight away from the body.
6. **Variation**—Using the same performance techniques, incline flyes are done on a 45-degree incline bench and affect the upper chest.

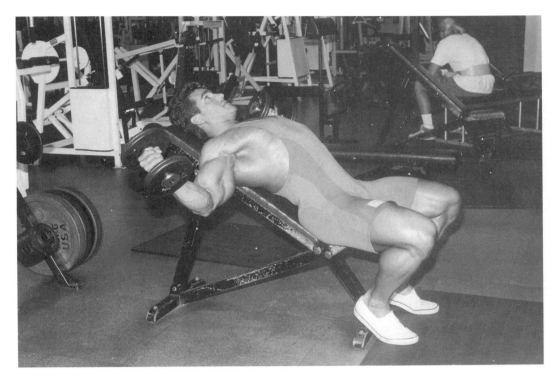

Flye stretch position (incline variation).

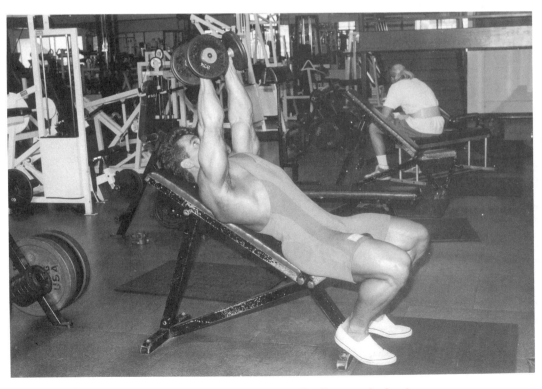

Flye contraction position (incline variation).

47

WIDE FRONT PULL-DOWNS

1. **Primary Muscle**—The back; mostly affecting width.

2. **Equipment**—A pull-down machine with changeable weights and a long bar attached to the pulley cable.

3. **Stretch**—You should be holding the exercise bar with an overhand grip that is eight to ten inches wider than shoulder width. The stretch is when your arms are fully extended and it feels as if your shoulders are dislocated upward and your lats stretched.

In an overhead grip, the palms face forward, away from the body. In an underhand grip, palms face up or toward the body.

4. **Contraction**—The arms are pulled all the way down so that the bar touches at mid to upper chest. The elbows should be kept pulled back on the same vertical plane as the hands and bar.

5. **Performance**—As described in Part One of "How the Muscles Work," from the stretch position you should first pull the shoulders down into their sockets and then continue to pull the bar down to the contraction point. It's important to keep the rib cage lifted and for the upper body to remain as upright as possible during the movement. Leaning the torso back changes the muscle focus of the exercise. Resist against the weight as the bar is returned to the stretch.

6. **Variation**—Wide-grip rear pull-downs use the same techniques, except that the bar is pulled behind the neck instead of to the chest. This exercise still affects back width, but focuses on the upper-back muscles. When first doing this movement, be careful to go slowly so that you don't hit your head with the bar. Lean your upper body slightly forward when doing rear pull-downs.

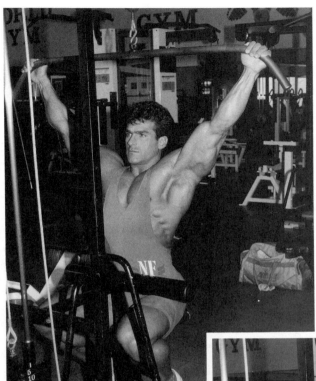

Wide Front Pull-down
stretch position.

Wide Front Pull-down con-
traction position.

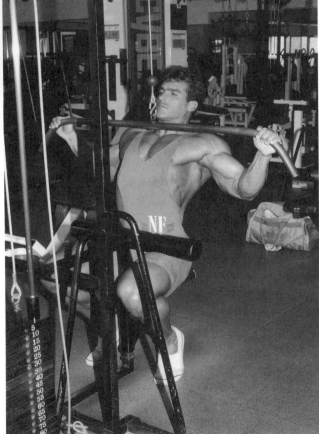

LOW-PULLEY ROWS

1. **Primary Muscle**—The back; mostly affecting thickness.

2. **Equipment**—A low-pulley machine with footrests to brace your body and a close-grip exercise handle. The handle should have a parallel or a slightly V-ed hand grip. If it is a V-ed grip, the narrowest part of the v faces top.

3. **Stretch**—Holding the handle, the arms should be stretched all the way forward and the upper body should be bent at the waist, stretching the back. The machine you use should allow you to fully stretch forward without the weights you are using touching the remaining weight stack. This is to maintain tension throughout the movement.

4. **Contraction**—The upper body should be upright and perpendicular to the ground. The arms should be pulled in until the handle touches just below the rib cage. The shoulders should be shrugged back and together. Keep the elbows close to the sides and pulled back as far as possible.

5. **Performance**—The upper body should move forward only far enough to allow a full stretch. No momentum is used to move the weights by bending and raising at the waist. Focus on making your shoulder blades squeeze together while raising the weight. Elbows are kept close in by the sides. The rib cage is raised and the back slightly arched during contraction, but this is not permission to lean the upper body back to add momentum.

6. **Variation**—None in apprentice routines.

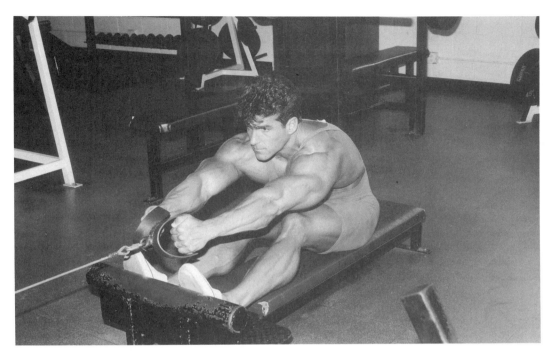

Low-Pulley Row stretch position.

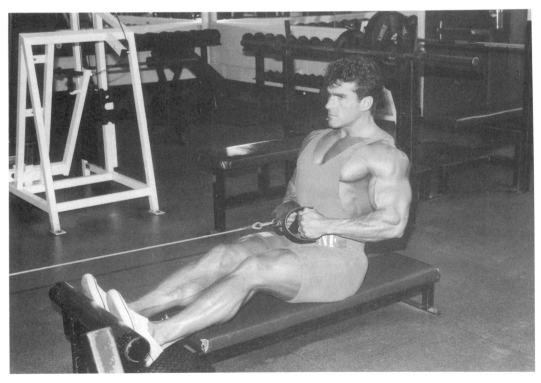

Low-Pulley Row contraction position.

BARBELL PRESSES BEHIND THE NECK

1. **Primary Muscle**—The shoulders; especially mid to front deltoid.

2. **Equipment**—A barbell and weights. An exercise bench with its back at a 90-degree angle to the floor (straight up and down). Some modern benches for shoulder pressing have weight stands attached.

3. **Stretch**—With an overhand grip and hands evenly spaced ten to twelve inches wider than shoulder width, the bar is lowered until it touches the base of the neck. Once again, the elbows are pulled back onto the same vertical plane as the hands and bar.

4. **Contraction**—Arms fully extended, elbows just a "hair" short of fully locking out. The shoulders should be down in their natural position and not shrugged upward with the bar.

5. **Performance**—Smoothly raise and lower the weight from stretch to contraction. Resist the weight as you lower it. Keep the rib cage *slightly* lifted, but the lower back should be pushed back into the bench.

6. **Variation**—Use the same performance techniques, holding one dumbbell in each hand. You may find two dumbbells harder to balance than a barbell; go slow and smooth and the balance will come after a few reps or sets. Raise and lower both dumbbells at the same speed. Palms still face forward.

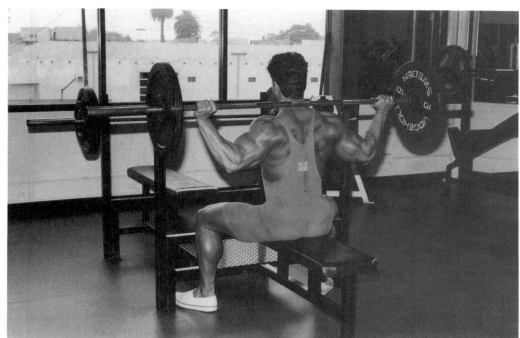

Barbell Press Behind the Neck stretch position.

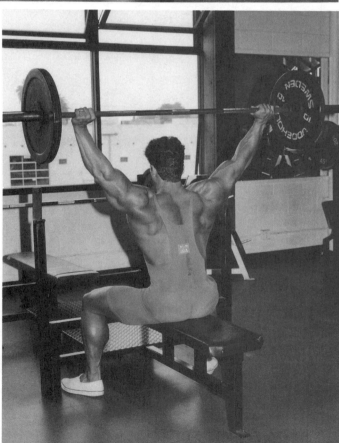

Barbell Press Behind the Neck contraction position.

DUMBBELL SIDE RAISES

1. **Primary Muscle**—Shoulders; especially side deltoid.
2. **Equipment**—Two dumbbells of the same weight.
3. **Stretch**—In the side raise, the stretch point happens when your arms are hanging down with the dumbbells right in front of your thighs and your palms facing each other.
4. **Contraction**—The dumbbells should be raised laterally until they are approximately at shoulder height.

**Dumbbell Side Raise
stretch position.**

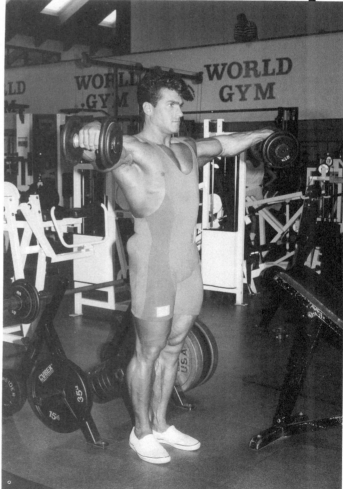

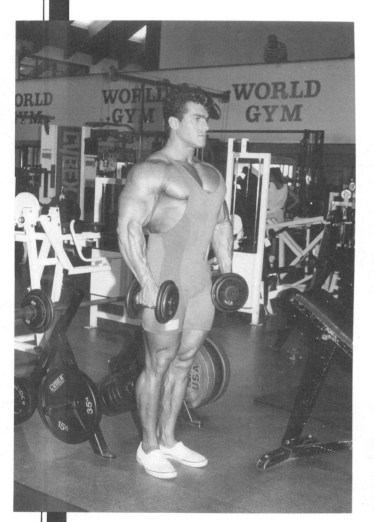

Dumbbell Side Raise contraction position.

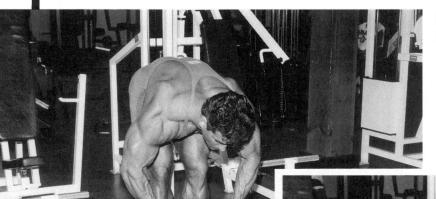

**Bent-over Dumbbell Side
Raise stretch position.**

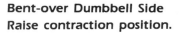

**Bent-over Dumbbell Side
Raise contraction position.**

5. Performance— At the bottom of the movement your palms should face each other. Your elbows should be, and remain, slightly bent. Raise your arms straight out to the sides (laterally) until the dumbbells are at shoulder level. Keep your torso upright. Don't swing the weights by bending and straightening at the waist, adding momentum. As you're raising the weights your palms will be facing the floor. When you get to the contraction, tip the dumbbell forward slightly—as if pouring water from a bottle. Don't shrug your shoulders up; keep them down in their sockets.

6. Variation—The key variation is a bent-over dumbbell side raise that targets the rear deltoid as its primary muscle. To do this exercise bend forward at the waist until your torso is parallel to the floor. Bend your knees some to make them act as shock absorbers. The movement is the same. The dumbbells hanging straight down is the stretch and the dumbbells raised laterally to shoulder level is the contraction. When performing this version keep your elbows out and in a lateral straight line with your shoulders. This keeps the movement focused on the rear deltoid instead of the back.

BARBELL CURLS

1. **Primary Muscle**—The biceps.
2. **Equipment**—A barbell and weights.
3. **Stretch**—Holding the bar with an underhand grip, the biceps are stretched when the arms hang down and the elbows are fully straightened.
4. **Contraction**—The bar is raised by bending the elbows. The biceps length is shortened and therefore flexed.
5. **Performance**—The upper arms should be kept as still as possible. The major action should come from the effort of bending and straightening the elbows. The bar is raised until the hands are palms inward, at approximately shoulder level. At this point the tip of the elbows should still be pointed down, toward the ground. The biceps should resist as the bar is lowered back to full stretch.
6. **Variation**—To perform incline dumbbell curls, you'll need two dumbbells and an adjustable incline bench at an angle of around 65 to 70 degrees. All the same rules apply. Arms hanging straight down is the stretch; elbows bent, dumbbells raised, upper arm stable and biceps flexed is the contraction.

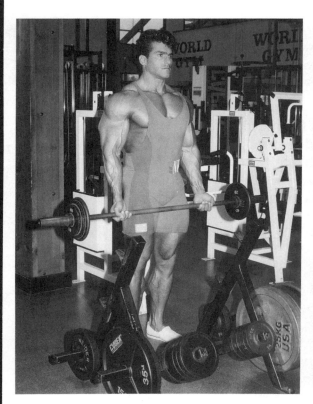 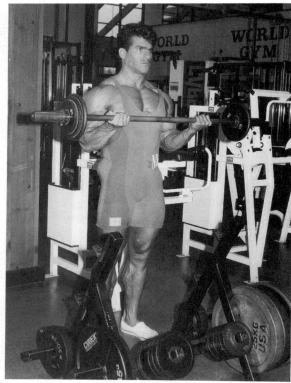

Barbell Curl stretch position.   **Barbell Curl contraction position.**

TRICEPS PUSH-DOWNS

1. **Primary Muscle**—The triceps.
2. **Equipment**—A high-pulley weight and cable machine with a medium-length straight bar.
3. **Stretch**—With the upper arms by the sides and torso upright, the elbows are fully bent and the forearms raised toward the biceps.
4. **Contraction**—The elbows are fully straightened and the arms are extended so that the hands and handle are nearly touching the front thighs.
5. **Performance**—You should raise and lower the forearms, hands and handle in a smooth, controlled way by bending and straightening the elbows. Use arm strength and not swaying or body momentum to move the weight.
6. **Variation**—On a flat exercise bench with a barbell or E-Z curl bar, lie so that your head is right at the end of the bench. Take a close overhand grip on the bar. The arms should be extended and the bar straight above your chest in the contraction position. Keep your upper arm in place and elbows pulled toward each other as much as possible. Now bend at the elbows and lower the weights to your forehead—that's the stretch. Raise the weight by flexing your triceps and straightening your elbows. This variation is called the lying triceps extension or lying French press.

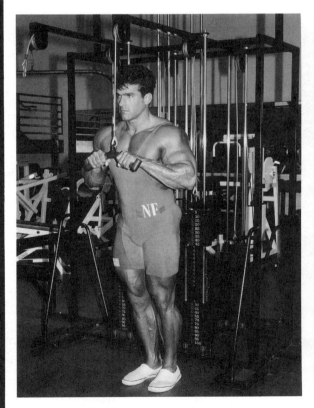

Triceps Push-down stretch position.

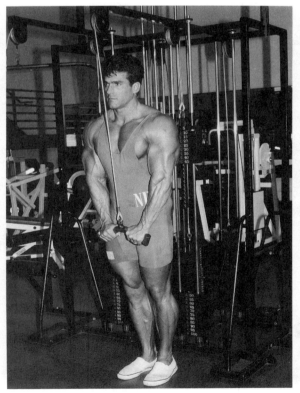

Triceps Push-down contraction position.

BACK SQUATS

1. **Primary Muscle**—The front thigh from the knee to the hips; also strongly works the hip and glute muscles.

2. **Equipment**—Barbell and weights, plus a weight stand, such as a squat rack, to rest the bar on.

3. **Stretch**—The knees and hip joints are bent and the butt is lowered from a standing position toward the floor.

4. **Contraction**—The knees and hip joints are straightened. The body is fully upright, with the legs straight.

5. **Performance**—Assume a solid stance with feet twelve to fifteen inches apart and toes pointed *slightly* outward. Evenly balance a bar across the base of your neck, with both hands holding on to the bar to assist in stabilizing it. Keep the chest out and eyes up at all times. Now do deep knee bends. You should bend your knees until your upper thighs go just below parallel to the ground. Keep your upper torso pulled back so that it remains as upright as possible. Do not bounce at the bottom or top of the movement; doing so could injure your knees.

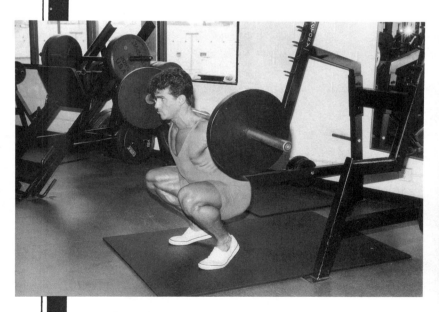

Back Squat stretch position.

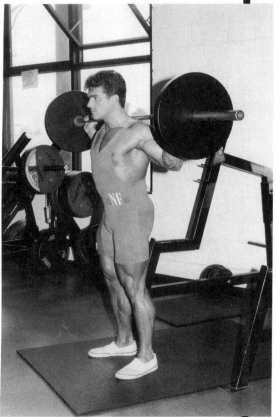

Back Squat contraction position.

6. Variation—The leg press involves the same principles of bending and straightening the knee and hip joints, but you do it seated in a machine. Let your legs lower until your thighs touch your chest and then squeeze the weight back to the top. Resist the weight and keep every rep under your control.

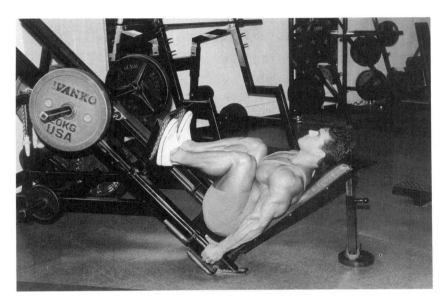

Leg Press stretch position.

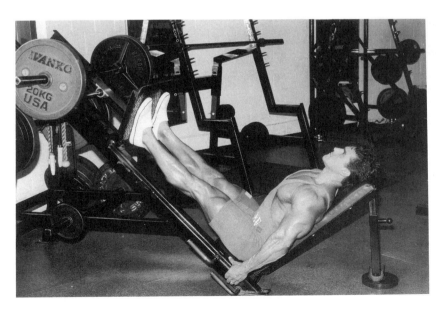

Leg Press contraction position.

LEG EXTENSIONS

1. **Primary Muscle**—Front thigh, from the knee to the hip.

2. **Equipment**—A leg-extension machine.

3. **Stretch**—The knees are fully bent while sitting on the machine. The feet are under the pads and pointed toward the ground.

4. **Contraction**—The knees are fully extended. The feet are extended out fully, forming a somewhat straight line between the hip, knee and ankle joints.

5. **Performance**—Adopt a smooth, controlled movement between contraction and stretch. Do not bounce the weight at either end of the movement. You can brace your body by holding the machine (it may have handles for this purpose) with your hands. Keep your torso upright and your hips and butt down and on the machine.

6. **Variation**—None in the apprentice routines.

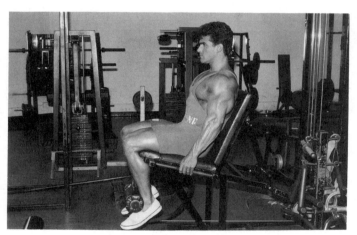

Leg Extension stretch position.

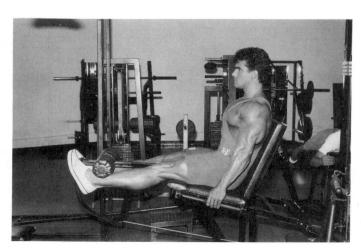

Leg Extension contraction position.

LYING LEG CURLS

1. **Primary Muscle**—The leg biceps (hamstrings) between the bottom of the glutes and the back of the knees.

2. **Equipment**—Leg-curl machine.

3. **Stretch**—You should be lying face down on the machine, with feet hooked under the pads and knees straightened.

4. **Contraction**—The knees are bent by pulling the feet toward the butt, shortening the length of the hamstrings.

5. **Performance**—Starting from the stretch, flex the hamstrings before even bending the knees. Now bend the knees and squeeze the weight up until the maximum contraction is found. Push your hips and butt forward (toward the bench) at the contraction point to further flex the leg biceps.

6. **Variation**—None for the apprentice routines.

Lying Leg Curl stretch position.

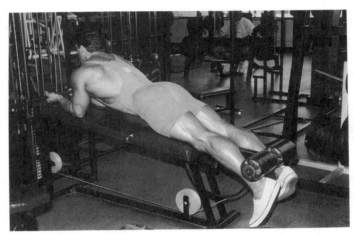

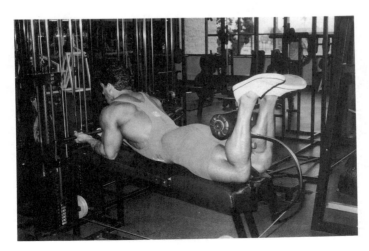

Lying Leg Curl contraction position.

61

STANDING CALF RAISES

1. Primary Muscle—The calf from the back of the knee to the top of the heel.

2. Equipment—An adjustable standing calf machine and a high block.

3. Stretch—The heels should be stretched as far toward the floor as possible, with the knees straight.

4. Contraction—The heels should be raised up as high as possible, with the knees straight.

5. Performance—Be sure to balance the weight on your shoulders so that your body is in a straight line up and down. Losing your balance or being unaligned could cause injuries at several points, including the lower back. Stand with the balls of your feet on the edge of a high block and three-quarters of your foot off the back. Simply bend at the ankle to raise and lower in order to contract and stretch.

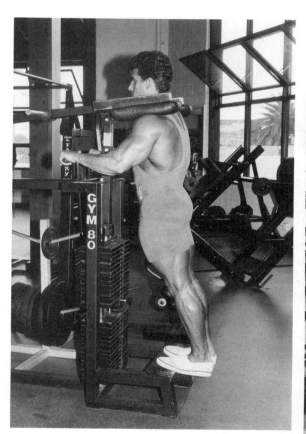

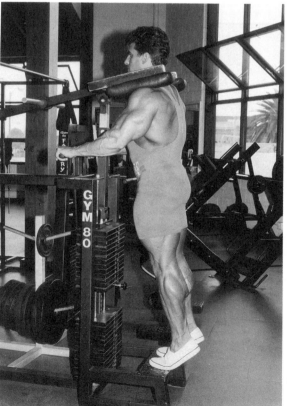

Standing Calf Raise stretch position.

Standing Calf Raise contraction position.

6. Variations—The two variations in your calf routines will be the leg-press calf raise and the seated calf raise. All the same rules apply to both. For the leg-press calf raise, you'll sit in a leg-press machine, with the balls of your feet resting on the bottom edge of the foot platform, and you'll raise and lower your heels. For the seated calf raise, use a seated calf machine. This means that you'll sit with your knees bent, once again raising and lowering your heels, but you'll be working the lower part of your calf, called the soleus, because of the bend at the knee.

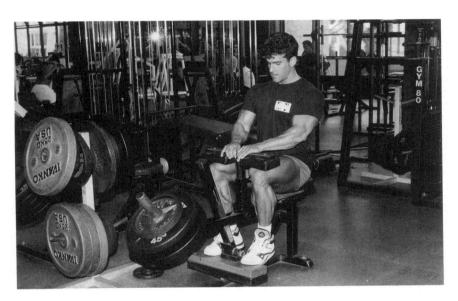

Seated Calf Raise stretch position.

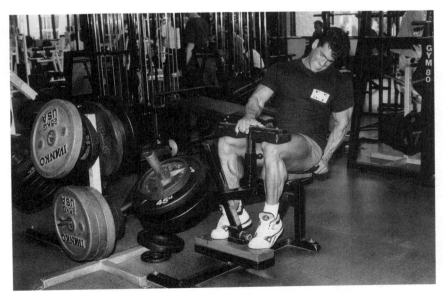

Seated Calf Raise contraction position.

CRUNCHES

1. **Primary Muscle**—Abdominals.
2. **Equipment**—None necessary; can, however, be performed lying on the floor with bent legs rested across a bench.
3. **Stretch**—the upper body should be lying flat on the floor.
4. **Contraction**—The upper body should be curled forward and the length between sternum and pelvis shortened.
5. **Performance**—Lying on the floor, bend your knees so that the upper leg is perpendicular to the torso and the lower leg is parallel to the floor. Push your lower back into the floor. Curl your chin forward until it is tucked into your collarbone (or near it). Now simply raise your shoulders off the ground and curl your head toward your knees, flexing your abs as you go. Return to the start. It is a small movement, but if you focus, it is physiologically the best and safest ab exercise.
6. **Variation**—None in the apprentice routine.

Crunch stretch position.

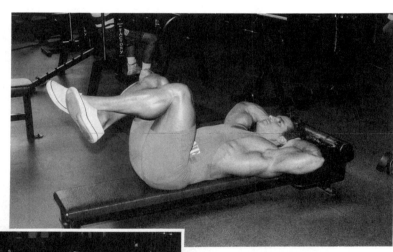

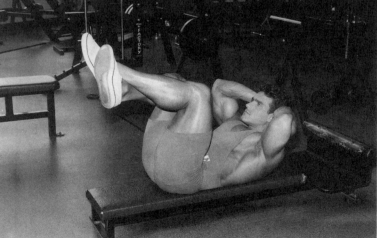

Crunch contraction position.

LYING LEG RAISES

1. **Primary Muscle**—Abdominals, with the emphasis on lower abs and hip extensors.
2. **Equipment**—A flat exercise bench.
3. **Stretch**—The legs should be lowered just below parallel to the floor.
4. **Contraction**—The legs should be raised about parallel to the floor.
5. **Performance**—Lying with your butt all the way to the end of the bench, extend your legs straight out. Keep both legs side by side and bend them slightly at the knees (keep them in this slightly bent position throughout). Moving only from the hip joint, raise and lower your legs. Push your lower back down into the bench and raise your head, curling your upper abs forward slightly. The best range of motion is six inches below parallel and ten inches above parallel to the floor.
6. **Variations**—Scissors are simply lying leg raises done one leg at a time. As one leg goes up the other comes down, like a swimming kick.

Hanging leg raises are done hanging from a pull-up bar. The stretch is your legs hanging down and the contraction is your bent knees raised above parallel to the floor.

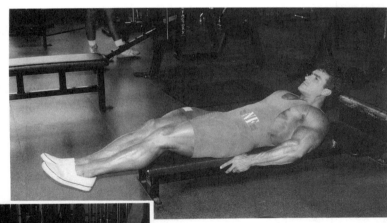

Lying Leg Raise stretch position.

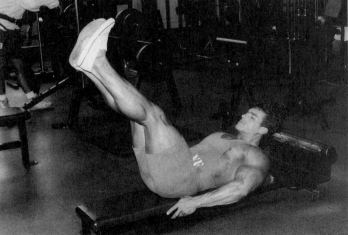

Lying Leg Raise contraction position.

BARBELL WRIST CURLS

1. **Primary Muscle**—The forearms.
2. **Equipment**—A barbell and weights; an exercise bench.
3. **Stretch**—The wrists should be bent backward, toward the floor, with the bar in both hands.
4. **Contraction**—The wrists should be bent (or curled) up until the muscles are shortened.
5. **Performance**—Rest the wrist joints just off the edge of a bench. Grab the bar with an underhand close grip (hands four to six inches apart). Hold your elbows together by wedging them between your thighs as you sit on the bench. Raise and lower the weight by bending the wrists in the appropriate direction.
6. **Variations**—The rules for the dumbbell wrist curl are the same, except that you stand up with your arms hanging by your sides and a dumbbell in each hand. Palms face your thighs. Bend your wrists in and out to do the reps. The wrist bending should be the only body movement.

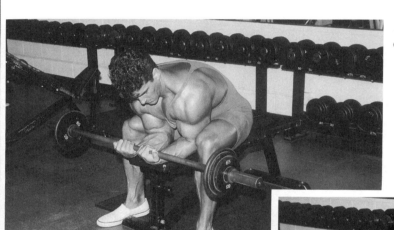

Barbell Wrist Curl contraction position.

Barbell Wrist Curl stretch position.

HYPEREXTENSIONS

1. **Primary Muscle**—Lower back, with the emphasis also on glutes and hamstrings.

2. **Equipment**—Hypertension bench.

3. **Stretch**—You should be fully bent forward at the waist and hip joint. The upper body should be lowered down and somewhat back toward the feet to maximize stretch.

4. **Contraction**—The body should be fully in line. You could, theoretically, draw a straight line from the ankles to the neck bisecting the knees, hips and shoulders.

5. **Performance**—The term "hyperextension" is a misnomer, because the lower back, especially in apprentice stages, should never be overextended backward. You should smoothly raise and lower your upper body by bending at the hip joint and focusing on flexing the lower back and butt muscles. Do not bring your torso above parallel to the floor.

6. **Variation**—None in the apprentice routines.

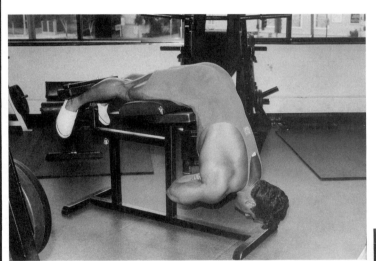

Hyperextension stretch position.

Hyperextension contraction position.

PART THREE: JOURNEYMAN AND MASTER EXERCISES

CHEST

Press Movements

Bench Presses
Incline Bench Presses
Incline Dumbbell Bench Presses
Flat Dumbbell Bench Presses
Dips
Push-ups

Flye Movements

Flat Dumbbell Flyes
Incline Dumbbell Flyes
Pec-Decks
Cable Crossovers
Cable Crossovers on Incline Bench

Pull-over Movement

Across-Bench Pull-over

PERFORMANCE TIPS

Chest Pressing: No matter what angle or pressing exercise I'm doing, I always begin the movement by first finding my correct body position. This is done by finding where the chest is most fully contracted (flexed) with the arms fully extended. Once I find that intense feeling, I mentally aim to duplicate it at the top of every single rep. It is essential to keep the elbows back on all press movements in order to maximize the muscle stretch. Even on dips, your elbows should be pointing out away from the body to keep the pecs as the primary muscle.

On barbell movements, touching the bar as high on your chest as possible also maximizes the stretch. Think of it this way—the greater the stretch, the greater the contraction.

On all pressing movements, you should lift your rib cage to put the pecs in their most efficient position, but don't arch your lower back and/or butt off the bench. This is extremely key on incline movements. If you lift your butt up off the bench on an incline bench press, you just turn it into a flat bench press and your upper chest will not be as effectively developed.

The exception to the rule of lifting the rib cage would be on dips done for the chest. On this exercise you should roll your upper body forward and touch your chin to the top of your chest to activate the pectoral muscles. Lifting the rib cage on this movement throws the primary work onto the triceps, which is great if that is the muscle you're trying to target. On dips for chest, your legs should also be forward, so that the side silhouette of your whole body would be almost a crescent moon shape.

Flye Movements: The key to flye movements is keeping the elbow-bending action to an absolute minimum. You want to function from the shoulder joint as much as possible. Just as with presses, you should keep your rib cage lifted and find the absolute perfect contraction on the first rep, then aim for its duplication on every one thereafter. Keep the elbows pulled back to increase the stretch. On dumbbell flyes and cable crossovers, your elbows should be pretty much kept bent at a 45-degree angle throughout the movement. On all press and flye movements, make sure your shoulders aren't pushed forward at the contraction point, in order to isolate the chest.

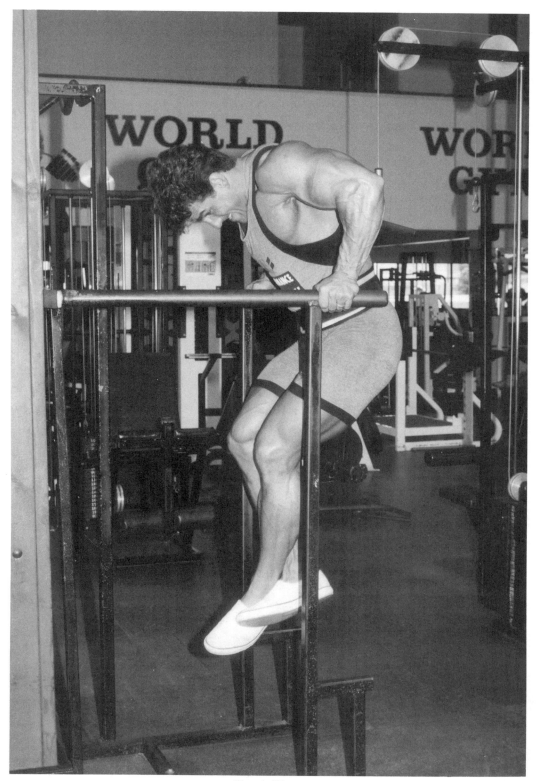

Chest Dips.

Pull-over Movements: The key to effective across-bench pull-overs is keeping your hips as low as possible throughout the movement, especially in the stretched portion, where the dumbbell is lowered back behind the head toward the floor. Keeping the hips low ensures maximum stretch. This exercise's greatest contribution lies in its tremendous stretch.

It is also important that the movement happen at the shoulder-joint rotation. This requires that you keep your elbows locked in a slightly bent position throughout the movement, in order to avoid activating the triceps. When you get to the top of the movement, squeeze your hands together (like the top of a flye) to flex the chest.

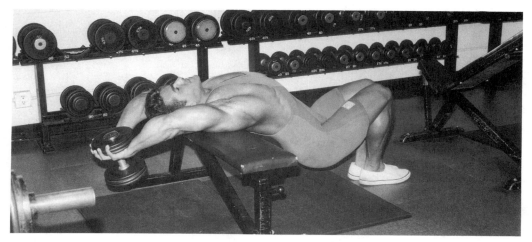

Across-Bench Pull-over stretch position.

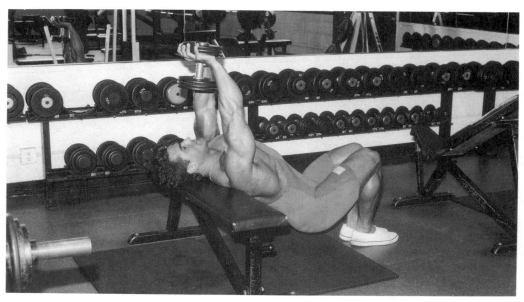

Across-Bench Pull-over contraction position.

BACK

Pull-down/Pull-up Movements

Wide Front Pull-ups
Wide Front Pull-downs
Wide Rear Pull-ups
Wide Rear Pull-downs
Close Grip Pull-downs
Medium-Grip Underhanded Pull-downs

Rowing Movements

Barbell Rows
T-Bar Rows
Low-Pulley Rows
One-Arm Dumbbell Rows
Two-Arm Dumbbell Rows

Shoulder-Rotation Movement

Straight-Arm Pull-ins

Shrug Movements

Barbell Shrugs
Dumbbell Shrugs
Half Deadlift/Shrugs

Lower-Back Movements

Half Deadlift/Shrugs
Hyperextensions
Good Mornings
Stiff-Leg Deadlifts (also listed as a leg-biceps stretching movement).

PERFORMANCE TIPS

Pull-down/Pull-up Movements: As described already in Part One of "How the Muscles Work," pull-down/pull-up movements consist of four key steps:

1. **Extending the arms fully to stretch the back.**
2. **Pushing the shoulders down into their sockets.**
3. **Pulling the bar down (pull-down) or the body up toward the bar (pull-up).**
4. **Returning to the stretch.**

Pull-downs and pull-ups affect the width of the back, but it is fallacious to assume that the wider your grip on the bar, the wider your lats will grow. On wide-grip movements, I usually hold the bar at a place where my hands are about six to eight inches wider apart than my shoulders. So if I hold my arms straight up in the air, I'll move my hands out six to eight inches wider to get the correct and most efficient width.

One thing that may help you focus on the contraction is picturing yourself actually pushing down against the force with your elbows.

On all front pull-downs/pull-ups, touch the bar at mid-chest and lift your rib cage to flex your lats.

Rowing Movements: Rowing generally affects the thickness of the back. That's because the nature of a row is to shrug the shoulder blades together. The one great caution that I make on rowing movements is to be overly watchful of your lower back. Barbell and T-bar rows, especially, place the lower back in an extraordinarily vulnerable position. Really focus in on making the form perfect on these movements, instead of on how much weight is slapped on the bar. On low-pulley rows, really let the weight stretch your lats out as you let your arms extend. Fight against the weight as you lower it by keeping your back flexed during the return from contraction to stretch.

Shoulder-Rotation Movements: The keys to the straight-arm pull-in are:

1. **Keeping your rib cage lifted.**
2. **Arching your back by sticking your butt out.**

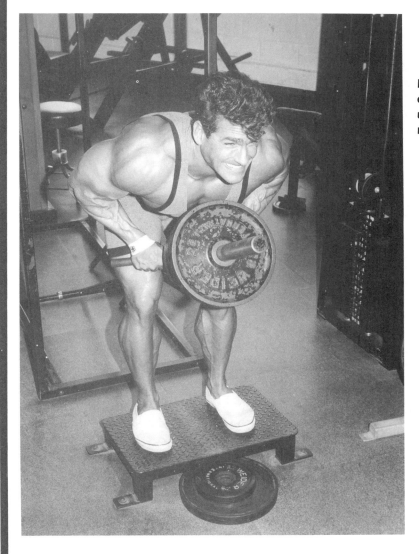

Remember to keep your chest out and eyes slightly upward when doing T-Bar rowing.

3. Allowing the rotation to happen only at the shoulder. Just like on the across-bench pull-over (these are physiologically fairly similar movements), it is important to keep the elbow joint stationary, in a slightly bent and locked position.
4. Allowing the lats to fully stretch at the extension of the movement.
5. Squeezing the bar toward the upper thigh and flexing the back for full contraction.

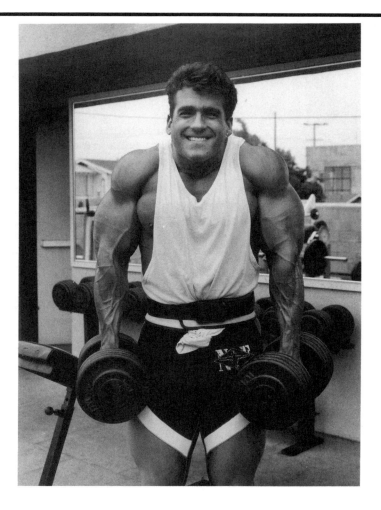

Dumbbell Shrug contraction position.

Shrug Movements: The most important thing to reinforce on shrugs is that the arms are only hooks that attach the body to the weight. They should not be muscularly involved in the movement, except in the sense of holding on to the weight.

The movement is simple. With your shoulders in their natural position, not forward or backward, the weight will give the stretch. To get to the contraction, just raise your shoulders toward your ears and then fight against the weight as you lower it back to the stretch. Make sure on all shrugging movements to get your body set before beginning the reps. It's sort of like how a golfer sets his or her body into position before beginning the swing. Never do the exercises "on the run" or you'll leave yourself open to injury.

The half deadlift shrug is a movement that works the entire spinal erector and trap system, from the top of the butt to the base of the neck. It is, as the name implies, a shrug with a half deadlift attached. Begin just as you would an ordinary shrug. Do a full rep, raising and lowering your shoulders (Position A). Then, when you get to the bottom of the stretch movement, bend at the waist and let the bar lower to just below your knees (Position B). Keep your back tight, your knees slightly bent and your body in a strong, solid position as you lower the weight. Lift the weight back up to the hanging-down arms, but body-upright position—the stretch position of an ordinary shrug (Position C). That is one rep. All the reps should be perfectly executed, under complete and deliberate control.

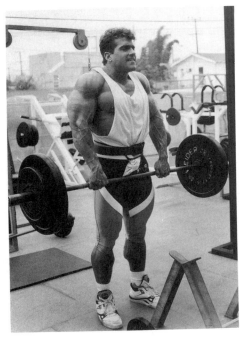

Half-Deadlift Shrug, Position A.

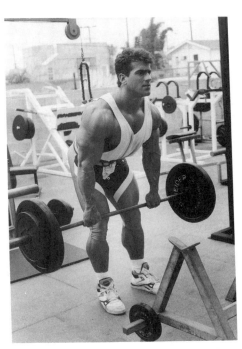

Half Deadlift/Shrug, Position B.

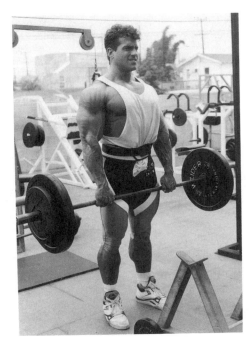

Half Deadlift/Shrug, Position C.

Lower-Back Movements: The lower back comes into play when the upper body bends forward at the waist. The key on hyperextensions and stiff-leg deadlifts is keeping complete control of the movement. You should stretch as far as your physiology will allow you to at the bottom of these movements (the half-deadlift shrug being the exception) and squeeze back to the contraction position by flexing the glutes, which will in turn flex the lower spinal erectors.

Because of the area's vulnerability to injury and its overuse in other body-part exercises (the lower spinal erectors are similar to the shoulders in their role of tying body parts together; thus both are susceptible to overuse injuries), the lower spinal erectors must be exercised with perfect form; attention to body alignment and full mental concentration are imperative.

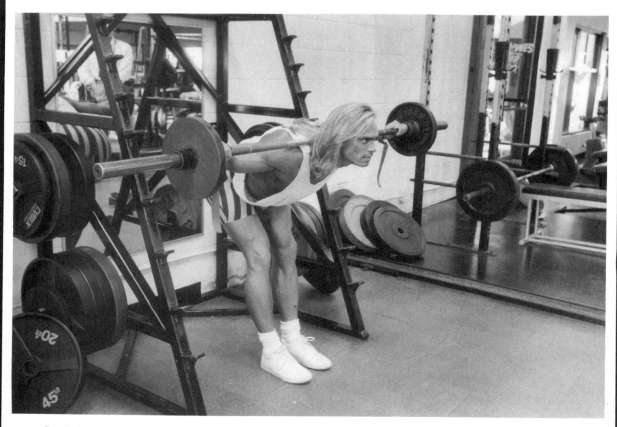

Rod Jackson performing Good Mornings. It is critical to keep your back straight, chest out and eyes up when executing this movement.

SHOULDERS

Pressing Movements

Barbells Behind the Neck
Dumbbell Presses
Alternating Dumbbell Presses

Lateral Movements

Dumbbell Side Raises
Bent-over Dumbbell Side Raises
Incline Side Raises
Lying Compound Side Raises
Reverse Pec-Decks
Rear-Pulley Crunches
One-Arm Pulley Side Raises
Bent-over Pulley Side Raises
Upright Rows

PERFORMANCE TIPS

Pressing Movements: The most effective tip I can give for shoulder-pressing movements is to not sacrifice the feel of the movement for the weight used. Once you are in touch with your muscles, you should be able to keep the delts flexed throughout the full range of motion. Don't just push the weight up and down. Experiment until you are able to find the absolute delt contraction at the top of a press. One key is keeping your elbows back throughout the movement. Also, don't arch your back and lift your rib cage on delt pressing. Arching will throw all the work solely onto the front delts. Push your lower back into the bench and roll your upper body *slightly* forward during the exercise to keep the whole muscle activated. Flex your rear deltoid during the stretch by pulling down on the bar and pushing your elbows back.

Think of pressing exercises as the exact opposite of pull-down movements for the back. Of course they work different body parts, but the stretch for pull-downs is the contraction position for delt pressing—and vice versa. Although this may not seem important, it's a reminder that your body is a whole and complete network, not just a bunch of unrelated body parts. Symmetrical development begins by understanding the interrelatedness of all the body's systems.

Lateral Movements: Because of the different angles that can be used, lateral movements offer an incredible amount of versatility in working shoulders.

Whenever I'm doing an exercise like dumbbell side raises, I'll begin the movement by first flexing the lateral deltoid head as hard as possible. It's the feeling of squaring off my shoulders and flexing the delts before the weight even moves. This motion will make the contraction at the top of the rep more complete and efficient.

Whether you're doing laterals or rear-deltoid side raises, you should only bring the dumbbells up high enough to squeeze the deltoid and not go past it. For example, when you do a dumbbell side raise the muscle is most flexed when the weights are at shoulder height. To raise them any higher would turn the movement into a trap exercise and take away from the tension on the lateral deltoid.

I classify upright rows as a lateral movement because the upper arm is moving in the same motion as in a side raise. While doing upright rows, it should feel as if you're squeezing toothpaste from a tube to get the contraction. Push outward with your hands as if doing a side raise. Your hands should not move on the bar; you should just be exerting pressure outward. This action, combined with squeezing the weight up, will increase efficiency dramatically.

Upright Row contraction position.

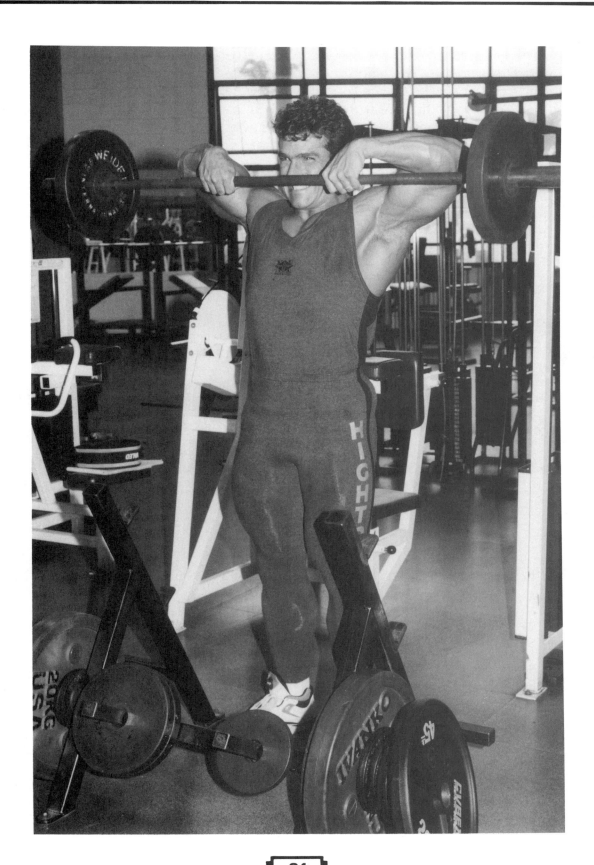

The lying compound side raise is a lateral movement that works the side and rear delt. You'll be lying on your side with the end of a bench in your armpit and one hand on the floor to brace your body. With a dumbbell in the other hand, you'll first lower the dumbbell in front of your body so that your elbow, wrist and hand fall into a straight line with your shoulder, perpendicular to your torso (Position A). Stretch all the way down, keeping your torso still, and squeeze the dumbbell back up along the same line it was lowered until it's right up over the side of your body (Position B). Then lower the dumbbell behind your torso (Position C) and squeeze it back up to the starting position. That's one rep. It's called compound because of its two-part nature. The part where the dumbbell goes out front works from mid to rear delt, and the part behind the torso works from mid to front delt.

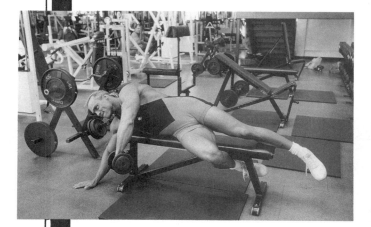

Lying Compound Side Raise, Position A.

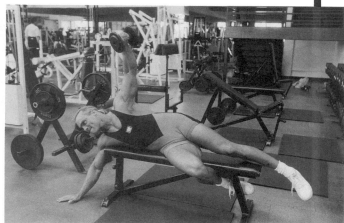

Lying Compound Side Raise, Position B.

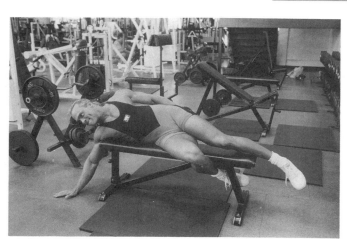

Lying Compound Side Raise, Position C.

BICEPS

Arm-Curling Movements

Barbell Curls
Barbell Preacher Curls
Two-Arm Pulley Preacher Curls
Two-Arm Pulley Curls
Incline Dumbbell Curls
Alternating Dumbbell Curls
Concentration Curls
One-Pulley Curls
One-Dumbbell Preacher Curls

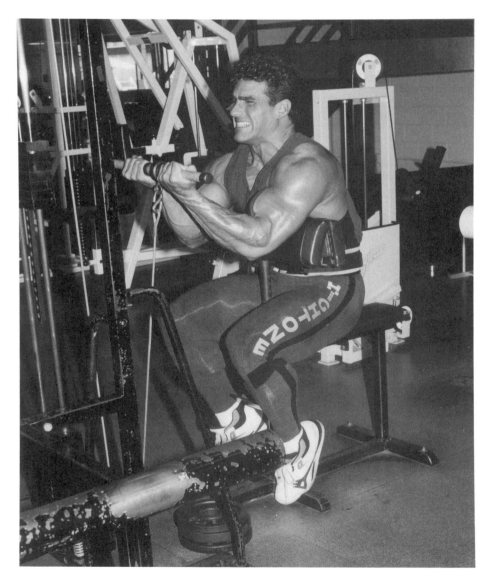

PERFORMANCE TIPS

Arm-Curling Movements: Two major factors come to mind in talking about biceps curls.

1. Making sure to fully stretch the muscle to full extension on every rep. Many people stop short and do only half or three-quarter reps on curling. You can make sure that you are getting that full stretch by flexing the *triceps* at the bottom (stretch) of each rep of curls. Remember the opposition of muscles: The triceps flex is the biceps stretch and vice versa.

2. Don't go past the point of greatest contraction at the top of a curl. For example, when I'm doing a preacher curl, there is a point at the top of the movement where the muscle is fully flexed but I can still keep moving the bar farther toward my body. That would be a mistake, because it would let up on the tension that's on the muscle and detract from its contraction. Focus in on finding the best contraction; it will be near the top of the movement, but don't be surprised if it's not at the farthest point that the weight can move.

TRICEPS

Pressing Movements

Bench Dips
Close-Grip Bench Presses
Dips for Triceps

Extension Movements

Push-downs
Reverse-Grip Push-downs
Rope Push-downs
Overhead Pulley Extensions
French Presses
Barbell Kickbacks
Two-Dumbbell Kickbacks
One-Arm Push-downs
Two-Arm One-Dumbbell Extensions

PERFORMANCE TIPS

Pressing Movements: The most essential element on triceps presses is keeping the contraction of the muscle focused into the meat of the triceps. As I discussed earlier, it is easy to "rest" the weight on your locked-out arms and avoid full contraction of the primary muscle. So you must really focus into the triceps and be sure to make bodily adjustments until you're able to flex the triceps fully on these movements. You'll know it when you find it, and once you find it you'll know you're cheating yourself by ignoring it. Focus also on keeping the force of the exercise, whether it's a dip or close-grip press, off the chest. This is a case where the arms should definitely be the driving force. Stretch your triceps fully at the bottom of the movement and begin the push toward the contraction position by flexing your triceps in the stretch position. This initiates the fibers and fires up the "mind to muscle-link."

Don't bounce the weights (whether it's your own body or a bar) on presses. The triceps attachments are a fragile group and can be susceptible to both ballistic and overuse injuries.

Extension Movements: On an exercise such as push-downs, you have a wide variety of different options to work with. Obviously, you can use different handles (straight bars, V-bars, ropes, etc.), but you can also perform the exercise in a couple of different ways. The first is the pure extension push-down. This is the exercise at its strictest. The upper arm should be kept stationary at the side of the body. The whole exercise revolves around raising and lowering the forearms, bending and straightening the elbows and stretching and flexing the triceps. Your general body position could best be described as upright, and the action focuses totally on the triceps.

The second push-down style turns the exercise into a combination pressing and extending movement. On this, you lean your upper body slightly forward. The pulley cable travels up and down pretty close to your body as you allow your elbows to go out wide, which will involve some shoulder-joint action. Then, from the stretch position (the hands up near the top of the chest and the elbows out wide), you push the weight back to the contraction position, as if doing a close-grip bench press. This is done by simultaneously straightening the elbows and pulling the upper arms back in toward the torso.

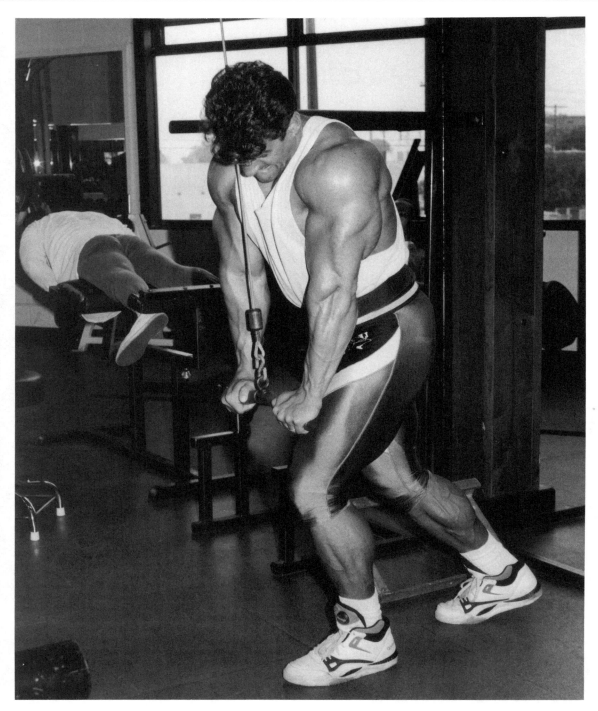

Note how the shoulders come into play in the Pressing Push-down.

The majority of the time I prefer the strict style, but put the "pressing" push-down in your routine now and then for variety.

Extension Movements

Leg Extensions
Sissy Squats

Pressing Movements
Back Squats
Front Squats
Leg Presses
Hack Squats
Lunges

PERFORMANCE TIPS

Extension Movements: The success of any single-joint extension movement definitely lies in its smooth transition from intense contraction to full stretch. It is important to get the full range of motion on leg extensions. The exercise called sissy squats is definitely misnamed—it is one of the most difficult and effective of all front-thigh movements. Generally, squats are classified as pressing movements, but sissy squats are effective because, when performed correctly, the hip joint is not activated in the movement; so they are, in theory, a knee-extension exercise. The key for this exercise is to lean the upper body back throughout the range of motion and to keep the hip joint straight. In other words, a relatively straight line should extend from your abdomen to your knees. Grab on to a stationary upright bar, go up on your toes with your feet close together, lean back and lower your body by bending at the knees until your knees touch (or come close to) the floor. Stand back up, taking your body along the same arc, and flex your quads and glutes as you get up to the top. Don't raise back up by duplicating a standard squat, in which the knees and hips are bent, or you'll lose out on the exercise's uniqueness.

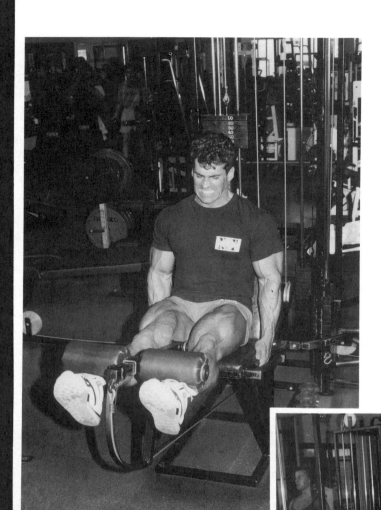

Performing a Sissy Squat.

Pressing Movements: The concept that escapes many people on leg presses, squats, etc. is that the exercises are much more than just raising weights up and down. If you aren't getting a hard flex at the top of each rep, you may be reducing the exercise's efficiency by 25 to 50 percent. When I do back squats, I focus on finding an intense front-thigh flex on every single rep and don't move on to a new rep until I've found it. This, of course, makes the exercise more difficult, but the results will be visibly apparent. Once you discover what an intense contraction feels like on a leg press (or any exercise, for that matter), you'll realize that you're cheating yourself whenever you avoid that feeling.

Be sure to stretch all the way down on your leg-pressing movements. Half and quarter squats are the surest way to screw up your knees, and bench squats, where you go down and bounce your butt off an exercise bench to prevent a full rep, should be banned from gyms worldwide. I have personally witnessed severe back and knee injuries resulting from this outdated technique. It would be far better to use less weight, do full reps and focus on the muscle. Injuries will only halt your progress.

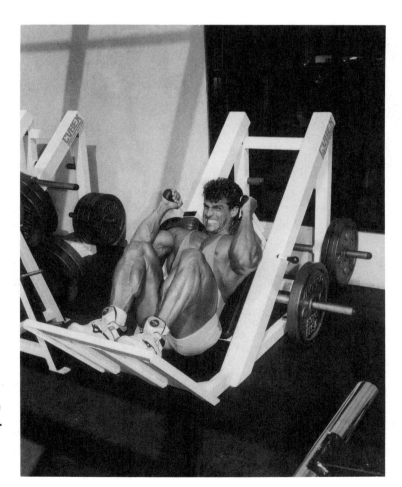

**Going for a full stretch
on the Hack Squat.**

LEG BICEPS

Curling Movements

Lying Leg Curls
Standing Leg Curls
Seated Machine Leg Curls
Dumbbell Leg Curls

Stretching Movements

Stiff-Leg Deadlifts
Hyperextensions

PERFORMANCE TIPS

Curling Movements: Follow the same rules here as with arm biceps:

1. Get a full stretch on every rep. Flex your front thigh if you're not sure where the full hamstring extension point is. Remember the opposition: The leg biceps' stretch is the front thigh's flex and vice versa.

You should also begin each rep by making sure your body is properly lined up and ready to go before starting. Flex the leg biceps in the stretch position and continue to flex harder and harder as you raise the weight to the contraction. When you get to the contraction point, push your hips forward to get the glutes out of the movement and to isolate and intensely contract the leg biceps. Then fight against the weight as you lower it back to a full stretch.

2. Do not go past the point of greatest contraction at the top of the movement. Just squeeze the weight up until you find the maximum flex and don't pull any farther. If you pull farther, you'll relax the hamstring and flex the glutes, losing your isolation of the primary muscles.

Stretching Movements: Stiff-leg deadlifts and hyperextensions work the entire muscle system from the top of the butt to the knees. By keeping the knees straight and bending forward at the hip joint, the hamstrings and glutes get tremendous stretch. You should lower your upper body forward until the hamstrings are maximally stretched and then squeeze back to the upright position by flexing the leg biceps and glutes. Only raise back to your natural posture on stiff-leg deadlifts and no higher than slightly above parallel to the floor on hyperextensions, in order to avoid jarring your lower erector muscles. I would caution you to do these movements slowly and with great contraction so as to avoid lower-back injuries. Trust me, it's completely possible to do very careful and very intense reps within the same set.

FOREARMS

Curling Movements

Reverse Curls
Zottman Curls

Wrist-Curling Movements

Barbell Wrist Curls
Dumbbell Wrist Curls
Reverse Barbell Wrist Curls
Pulley Compound Wrist Curls (a bi-set of two-arm pulley wrist curls and two-arm reverse-pulley wrist curls)

PERFORMANCE TIPS

Curling Movements: These movements follow all of the same rules that apply to biceps curling with two exceptions:

1. Reverse curls are done with the palms facing down when the arm is in the contraction position.

2. Zottman curls are done with the palms facing in toward each other throughout the movement.

All of the same principles of full stretch and full contraction must still be respected.

Wrist-Curling Movements: No matter if you're working the palm side or the back-of-the-hand side of your forearms, wrist curls are versatile enough to help you accomplish your goal.

Barbell wrist curls are usually done palms up, with the hands, wrists and bar hanging off the end of a bench. Reverse barbell wrist curls would be just the opposite: The palms face down. This is another example of opposition muscles—one side's flex is the other side's contraction. An exercise I call a pulley compound wrist curl is one that works the forearms from both angles in a bi-set fashion. I sit on the floor, use a low pulley and medium-length bar (preferably with a handle that rotates) and start with palms-up wrist curls to "positive failure" (the point at which I can do no further reps without compromising form) and then immediately switch to palms-down wrist curls. It's a very effective compound movement.

ABDOMINALS

Crunching Movements

Crunches
Twisting Crunches
Frog Kicks

Leg-Raise Movements

Lying Leg Raises
Hanging Leg Raises
Scissors

PERFORMANCE TIPS

Crunching Movements: As I discussed in Part One, the whole point here is to shorten the distance from the pelvis to the sternum. Your lower back should be pushed down into the bench or floor on crunches. Be sure to make the movement sure and "squeezy" instead of throwing your body. If you put your hands behind your head, don't pull too hard with them or you could wind up with a strained neck. Control, flex and stretch. For twisting movements, aim your right elbow toward your left side and vice versa. The twist does not need to be exaggerated to be effective—*if* you use the muscle, and not momentum to crunch your abs.

Leg-Raise Movements: In the lying leg raise, you should raise your head and tuck your chin into your chest to activate the abs. Next, raise and lower your legs from the hip joints, flexing the lower abs throughout the range of motion. The secret to finding your lower abs is pulling in on the muscles just above your hipbones. Breathe out and pull in. Now push out against those muscles, but don't stick your belly out—just push as if against an immovable wall. Keep this taut feeling as you lower and raise your legs.

CALVES

Heel-Raise Movements

Standing Calf Raises
Seated Calf Raises
Leg-Press Calf Raises
Donkey Calf Raises

Tibia Movement

Tibia Raises

PERFORMANCE TIPS

Heel-Raise Movements: On these movements, the more locked you keep the knee joints, the higher toward the knee you'll work the calf muscles. This is why seated calf raises work lower calves and standing calf raises are considered an upper-calf movement. The fundamental secret to calves lies in the stretch. Calf muscles are extraordinarily dense muscle fibers that are very compactly formed. Because of this you should focus not only on a full stretch at the bottom of the exercise, but also stretch your calves on a high block in between sets. Calves respond very well to what would generally be considered very, very high reps. I've recommended intense sets of fifty to seventy reps, combined with intense stretching, for athletes who can't get their calves to respond to traditional methods. I consider the twelve-to-fifteen-rep range to be low for calves, fifteen to twenty-five reps to be medium, and twenty-five to seventy to be high. Remember to adjust your perspective according to the specific needs of each body-part system.

Tibia-Raises: I work the front of my calves (the tibias) by placing my heels on a high block with three-quarters of the foot extended forward of the block. The exercise simply involves lowering the toes toward the ground to stretch the muscle and raising them back up to flex it. The tibia and the muscles surrounding the shin are the opposition group to the gastronemius and soleus. Tibia raises are important in balancing strength and development, both physically and visually, in the overall calf-muscle system.

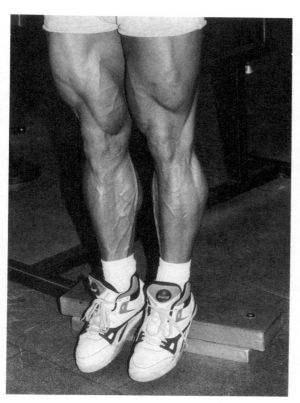

Tibia Raise stretch position.

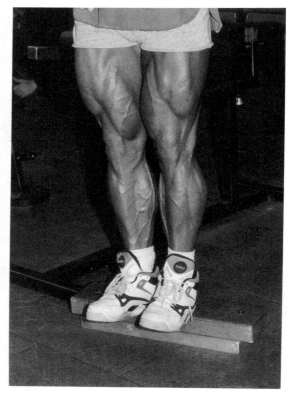

Tibia Raise contraction position.

Stretching and Aerobics

Besides weight training, are there any other physical activities that will help you attain physical flawlessness? My emphatic answer is yes! Your weight training is going to be the most efficient way for you to sculpt your muscular structure, but those exercises alone will not cover the full spectrum of whole-body fitness. Let's take a look at two areas of physical activity that, when properly used, will not only assist you in achieving your weight-training goals, but can become integral parts of your fitness strategy.

The first is stretching and the second is aerobics. In the same way there is a right way to do your weight exercises, there is also a correct way to use stretching and aerobics in your program.

I'm also a perfectionist when it comes to proper use of both of these activities. You want to enhance your chances of reaching your goals with everything you do in the gym. Because yours is a ten-week goal, you want everything to work as quickly and efficiently as possible. Striving for perfection is going to be the key to achieving this efficiency. You don't have any time to waste during the next ten weeks; you need to do things the right way from the very beginning.

When I was younger and just beginning to train, many coaches and sports "experts" were still telling athletes that they should be very cautious with bodybuilding-type training. The logic was that athletes would become "muscle-bound" and wouldn't be able to touch their own noses due to tight, overdeveloped muscles.

The real experts knew then (as has since been documented) that weight training would enhance an athlete's performance as long as the workouts were tailored to the sport. The term "sport-specific" was developed, and it meant that training had to revolve around activities that mimicked the demands of a particular sport. If you wanted to be a champion runner, you had to train like a runner. The weight workout you did had to be designed to enhance the particular strengths that a runner needed.

I feel that the "muscle-bound" mythology can be chalked up to a couple of factors. The first is the mistaken notion that all weight-training routines are the same. The second is the look of athletes involved in sports whose key skill developer is systematic weight training.

If you look at a still photo of a competitive bodybuilder, for example, you might assume that he is very "stiff" and unflexible because of the pose he is in. But posing is only done as a way to best display an athlete's physical development; it's not indicative of flexibility. In fact, many of the top professional bodybuilders I know are *very* flexible, and must be in order to efficiently work at their sport.

While research has so far shown no connection between the relative "tightness" of a muscle and its development, I've found that there is a very definite connection. I achieve the best gains in body parts that are flexible and supple. When a muscle is unflexed (relaxed), you should be able to sink your finger down into it. I'd bet that if a *relaxed* muscle is hard to the touch, it is, in most cases, a stubborn body part.

In order to avoid a tightness in the muscles, a good stretching routine needs to be incorporated into your overall regimen. Stretching your muscles provides a great way to warm up your body prior to a workout. Extra caution must be used, though, when stretching "cold" muscles. Have you ever used a rubber band on a really cold day? It's real brittle, right? Your muscles are kind of like rubber bands. What would happen if you were to suddenly pull that cold rubber band taut? Chances are it would break. You could keep the band from breaking by gently warming it up, stretching it a bit at a time until its flexibility returned. Your muscles warm up in a similar way. If you're warming up by stretching, take it slow and easy. Stretching should always be done slowly, smoothly and under complete control. Ballistic or bouncing stretches can and will lead to injuries ranging from minor to severe. Your ten-week program can quickly be derailed by a muscle pull or any structural injury.

My personal experience with stretching has always been very good—as long as I took it slow and easy. The one exception happened several years ago. I was warming up my thighs and hamstrings prior to a leg workout, but I was in a bit of a hurry. I only had one hour to warm up, do my workout, shower and rush to a business meeting. In my rush I got sloppy with my stretches, bouncing in them, thinking that I could warm up faster. I was really flexible at the time and feeling invincible. I went into a full split and then tried quickly to touch my forehead to the leg extended out front. As soon as my head touched my knee I felt a *pop*. I not only felt it, but I thought I heard the noise echo through the gym—even though it was only inside my head. The back of my leg tingled with intense numbness and then more intense pain. I had severely pulled my hamstring. Even with ice, massage, ultrasound and every type of therapy, my leg training was set back well over a month. It served as a tremendous lesson. I would never make the mistake of bouncing while stretching again. It was my first major training injury, and taught me that my body was not made of steel. If I wanted longevity as an athlete, I was going to have to respect my body's limits and train smarter than ever.

Besides just warming up the muscles, stretching can be used to cool down at the end of a weight workout. There is also a current theory that stretching the body part being worked in between sets of exercises will allow greater development to take place. There is nothing wrong with this theory. In fact, I've seen athletes make slightly faster gains in lagging body parts when they stretch a muscle between sets of exercises where the body part is isolated.

It goes back to what I said earlier about hardness vs. suppleness in a body part in relation to its ease of development. The stretching is done mainly to coax these hard, tight places into greater flexibility. The resulting suppleness allows blood and nutrients to travel more freely in and out of the muscle. When this occurs, greater development can take place.

STRETCHING

The point of stretching is to elongate the muscles, so I want you to think in terms of lengthening. Everything about how you stretch should be smooth, slow and long. When you move into a stretched position, you should extend the muscles being stretched until they are taut. Hold that position for a few seconds, then stretch just a bit farther and hold that position for twenty to thirty seconds. You will not be getting the full benefit if you move into a stretch, hold it for four or five seconds and move out. Many people tend to get impatient when stretching. You just have to take deep breaths and be patient. Hold your stretches, and *don't bounce*. Watch how a cat stretches its body. Think of yourself as a big cat moving with purpose and hidden power into each stretch position. If you are just starting out and feel inflexible, take your time. It took you years to get this stiff; surely you can give yourself a couple of weeks to get your limberness back. Be especially careful around any injured areas like lower back, knees, etc. If you have in the past or are now being treated for injuries in any of these vulnerable areas, consult your doctor for advice.

In my stretching routine I use five different core stretches and slight variations of each one to work on key body areas.

Chest Deltoid Biceps Stretch: Depending on your hand placement, you can emphasize either the chest or biceps on this stretch; you'll be stretching the front deltoid in both positions. This one is done one side at a time. Give equal energy to each side on any one-sided stretches.

Place your hands against a stationary object. It could be a wall, a doorway or a vertical bar on a piece of gym equipment. Your arm should be straight and your shoulder pushed down in its natural position. To stretch your chest, rotate your arm so that your palm faces forward and your elbow points down. For the biceps, rotate your arm so that your palm faces down and your elbow points back.

Hand height can vary between just above and just below shoulder level. The higher your hand is placed, the lower the area of your chest that you stretch. Putting your hand below shoulder level stretches the upper chest. With your arm straight and hand in the desired position, gently rotate your body *away* from your outstretched arm until you feel tension in your chest or biceps. Hold the stretch; release slowly and switch sides.

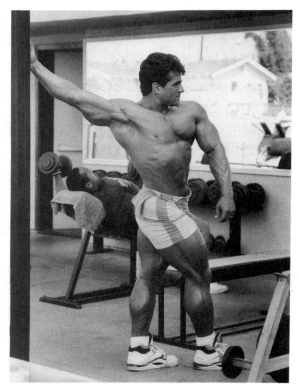

Chest/Deltoid/Biceps Stretch.

Back Stretch: This routine, also done one side at a time, will stretch the entire back, from upper to lower. Use a vertical upright bar on a piece of gym equipment. Pick a machine that's bolted down so it won't move when you pull against it. Stand so that the bar you grab is right at your side. If you are going to stretch your left side, the bar should be on the right and your right foot should be placed next to it. Stand with your feet about two to three feet apart. With your left arm outstretched, bend and rotate your body so that you grab the bar with your left hand, just above your right foot. You will feel the stretch in your back. To intensify the stretch, pull your upper body away from the bar while still holding on. You can make the stretch even more intense by pushing your body away from the bar with your free arm. You should be hanging on with your left and pushing away with your right and vice versa. You'll need to bend your knees to get into the position. If you straighten your knees while you're stretching your back, the hamstring will also get a stretch.

Go slow at first. If you can't grab the vertical bar down by your foot, start with a higher position and work your way down as you become more flexible.

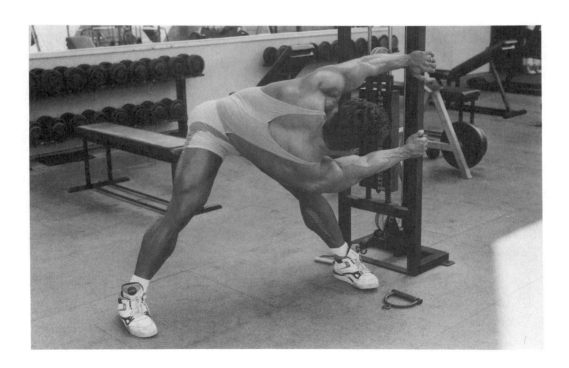

Back Stretch.

Hamstring/Lower-Back Stretch: This stretch has many different variations. I've illustrated a standing one-leg hamstring stretch. Place the foot of the outstretched leg on a solid support at about waist level. Make sure you have your balance on the leg you're standing on. Keep your knee completely straight on your outstretched leg. Grab the ankle or foot with both hands. Keep your back straight and bend at the waist and hip joint. Push your chin way out front and go out and forward, trying to place your head on your foot. Yes, it's physically impossible. Your chin will actually go to your knee, but I want you to really elongate forward as you bring your upper body down. Use your hands to *gently* pull your upper body into the stretch. Hold and then switch legs. A good variation of this stretch is sitting on the ground with both legs straight and V-ed out at a 90-degree angle. Use the same stretching technique as above, but keep the opposite leg straight at all times. Keep both knees locked to maximize the hamstring and lower-back stretch. Notice the similarity between this stretch and the stretch position for hamstring exercises. In fact, all the stretches in this section replicate exercise stretch positions.

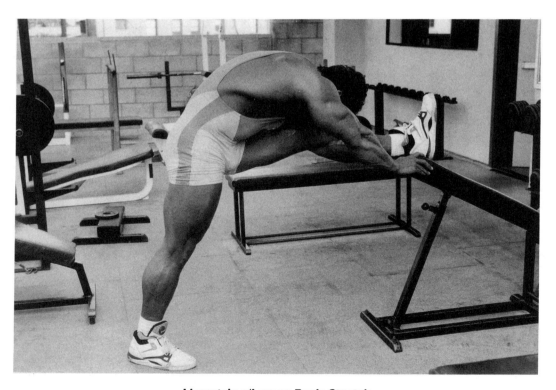

Hamstring/Lower-Back Stretch.

Front-Thigh Stretch: For this section I try to find a support that is about waist-high, like the top of an incline bench or the weight bar on a 45-degree leg press. Face away from this support, bend your knee and carefully hook the top of your foot on whatever you're using as support. You should immediately feel the front thigh stretch, just from having your knee bent so much. If you have any knee problems at all, go *very* slowly on this stretch. If you have any pain besides a taut feeling in the muscle—stop. To intensify the stretch, lean your upper body back. To further intensify, slowly move your knee back, increasing the tautness in the muscle. Come out of the position slowly and switch legs.

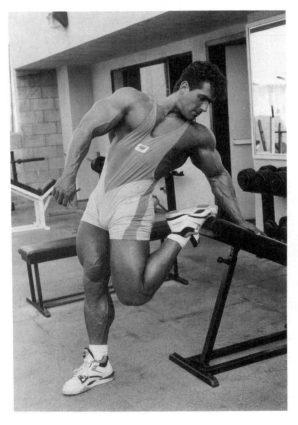

Front-Thigh Stretch.

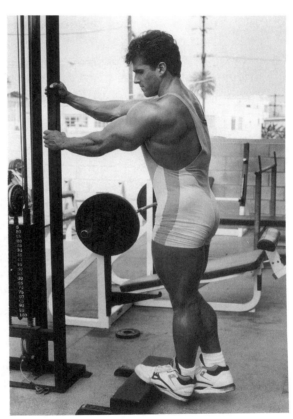

Calf Stretch.

Calf Stretch: This stretch directly duplicates the stretch position on a calf-raise exercise. Stand with your toes and the ball of your foot on the edge of a high block. Simply let your body weight stretch your heel to the floor until there's tension in the calf. I like to do this one leg at a time for a better stretch. If your heel touches the ground, you'll need a higher block. You can also use a step, like on a staircase. Keep your knees straight and don't bounce.

AEROBICS

Whereas training with weights builds the strength of skeletal muscles, aerobic exercise builds the strength of the cardiovascular system. In order to have complete fitness, you must engage in both forms of exercise. Recent research shows that each type of exercise covers gaps in the other's "total fitness" efficiency. You'll get some degree of cardiovascular fitness from an intense weight workout, but not to the extent that you'll get when performing a continuous movement in order to maintain your heartbeat within a target range. Weight-training workouts have a start-and-stop element to them; you perform a set and then take a short rest before doing the next one. The pulse rises dramatically during the exercise and decreases during the pause between sets. If you were to perform an endless cycle of weight exercises (moving, with no rest, from one exercise to another), a major limitation would present itself. Unless you were highly skilled and conditioned for this type of routine, you would run out of steam after a very short time and would fully stimulate neither muscular nor cardiovascular development.

There are people who do rely on circuit training (doing one set each of, say, ten different exercises with no rest in between) for their fitness goals. The majority of people using circuit-training routines are looking for a way to spend very little time training and aren't concerned with making their bodies look flawless. While some people do get desirable results from this training style, it still has limitations. Also, many experts agree that full cardiovascular development occurs only after twenty to thirty minutes of sustained exercise that keeps the heart rate at a target level. Most people doing a circuit-training routine still stop and rest after a circuit is completed, so the heart rate drops. Exercises are rarely taken to intense positive failure on circuit-training routines, and therefore full muscular development is not possible.

There is a routine that I have experimented with that uses circuit training as its model. It combines a full-body circuit of two exercises per body part with substantial exercise poundages, high repetitions, positive failure and no rest at any point during the circuit until thirty to sixty minutes (depending on conditioning) of the routine have been performed. This is one killer workout. When I tried it, I considered myself to be in very good muscular and cardiovascular condition. I not only dropped from exhaustion after thirty minutes, but I didn't recover for a week and I became physically ill at the thought of going through it again. I mean, I love to train hard, but this was *the* hardest thing I'd ever physically put myself through.

It is far more efficient to separate the two types of workouts and get the most from each. Your most intense workout should be the weight training. Aerobic exercise should be done only with enough intensity to place and hold the pulse rate in the target range. It should not be a "muscular" workout. Don't be like the bodybuilder who, after I commented that his physique would benefit from some aerobics, went over to the stationary bike, got on and cranked the tension up as high as it would go. He lasted about three minutes, getting a tremendous pump in his front thighs but doing nothing for his cardiovascular system or metabolism. Don't approach aerobic exercise like you're doing a maximum set of squats, where you're proving how strong you are. In fact, if you're feeling too much muscle burn when doing aerobics, you're probably at too high an intensity.

Aerobic exercise not only improves your lungs and heart, it also helps you create a more efficient metabolism. This is especially important when someone is first starting to work out. I always recommend aerobic workouts to apprentices whether they're trying to gain or lose weight. Aerobic conditioning will benefit weight workouts and vice versa, just by getting the whole system into better overall condition.

TARGET HEART RATE

Your week-by-week programs will tell you what your target pulse rate should be and how long each aerobic session should last. Your target heart rate is calculated by first subtracting your age from 220; for example, if you are 30, your maximum heart rate would be 190. Then take 75 percent of that figure, or 142.5. You would want to maintain somewhere around 143 beats per minute during the entire duration of an aerobic activity.

Calculate your target pulse range according to the percentage given in your program. You should increase or decrease exercise intensity to keep your pulse in its target range.

TYPES OF EXERCISES

My favorite aerobic exercise is the stationary bike. I also use a stair-climbing machine and fast walking in order to add variety to my workouts. I'd suggest using one or more of these types of exercise. Remember that target heart rate and not muscular burn is the goal here.

Stationary Bicycle: This machine is superior to outdoor cycling because there is no stop and start, like stopping for lights, etc. A relatively low tension should be used with a fast-pedal R.P.M. Use smooth, even pedal strokes to prevent knee trauma. The seat height should be adjusted so that when the pedal is closest to the floor, the knee is just short of locking out. Some people get numbness in the genital area when biking. A special split-seat has been developed that has a gap running down the middle to help with this problem. Some find that padding the seat with a folded towel also helps.

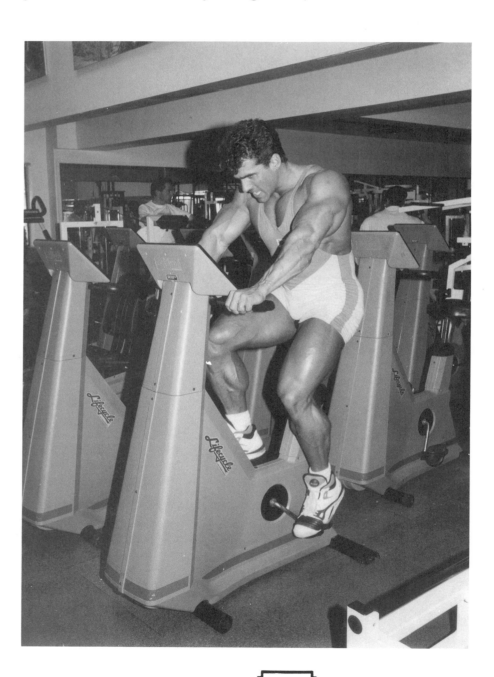

Stair-Climbing Machine: You must be very cautious using this device not to bounce as you step up and down. Ballistic knee injuries are quite common among bodybuilders using stair machines. A lot of the machines have some "play" at the bottom of the step, and there is the temptation to bounce out of this bottom part in the belief that you are working harder. Be careful. Correctly used, stair climbing is a great aerobic activity.

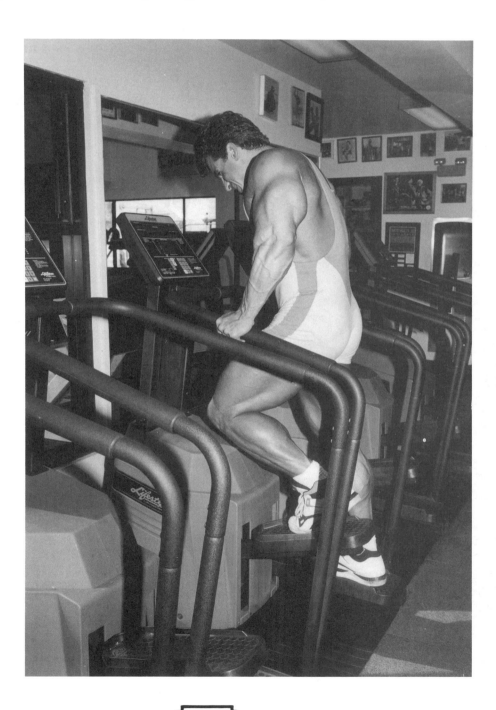

Fast Walking: This is a tremendous and often overlooked exercise. The best thing about fast walking is its relatively low impact on feet, knees and lower backs—the key injury areas for runners. I find that although it takes a few minutes to get my pulse into target range, I can get as much out of this as jogging and avoid possible injuries. To make walking a really effective aerobic conditioner, you can't just stroll along, window-shopping. Move along at a *very* fast walking pace to get your pulse up and then adjust your pace to keep it there. The best thing about walking is that you can do it practically anywhere. So if you're traveling and can't find a bike or stair climber, get out and hit the pavement or the trail.

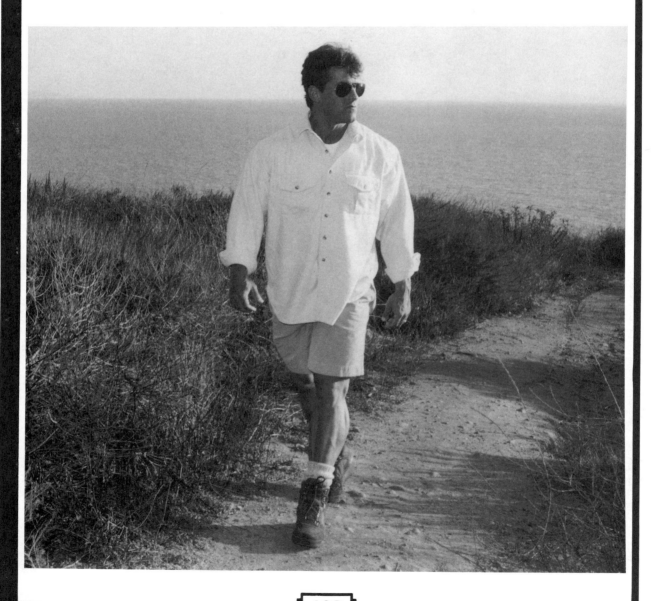

The Apprentice Program: Introduction

Welcome to the apprentice section of the book. You might be wondering why I didn't just call this a beginner's section. Why "apprentice"? The answer is that I see your flawlessness goals as akin to learning a craft. In your quest to become a craftsman, you'll travel through three stages of exercise skill: apprentice (beginner), journeyman (intermediate) and master (advanced).

This book is filled with information that will help you make sense of what may very well be brand-new to you. You'll be doing mental and physical exercises that will give new meanings to workouts, food and self-image. In the introduction to this book I touched very briefly on the ten elements that I felt were needed to build and keep a flawless body. Each of the following chapters take their respective themes from these elements. Preceding each week's workouts are tips, suggestions and assignments designed to make this program more effective for you. I also want you to turn to "Eating Right" in the Appendix and select the eating plan that best suits your individual needs.

The reason I separated the workout and nutrition sections is because of each individual's different needs. For example, you may be an apprentice in the gym, but need to gain weight. Your training program would be the same as someone wanting to lose weight, but your nutrition strategy would be different. Of course, you *will* find general nutrition information in each of your ten workout chapters. This information applies no matter what nutrition plan you're following. You should give equal emphasis to both your workouts and your eating schedules.

There is also a section in the book's Appendix that offers hints on how you can improve your nonmuscular appearance. It only makes sense that if you're busting your butt to achieve flawlessness and doing the nutritional stuff to back it up, you'll also want to pay attention to complexion, hair etc. So in that section I've included some simple and basic grooming tips.

The workout program has been designed so that week by week it grows slightly more intense and challenging. You may not notice the additional challenges because your body will be adapting and your self-esteem will be climbing. If you take a look in the mirror, though, you'll see how well the program works.

There's also a sort of "early-promotion plan" in this program. If you find that you're adapting so rapidly to the workouts that you don't feel fully challenged, you'll have the chance, at any point past four weeks, to promote yourself up to the Journeyman Program. I must caution you to evaluate yourself as objectively as possible before moving up, though. If you move up and haven't fully done your homework, you'll pay the price. I've included a checklist of questions in Week Five's chapter to help you determine how to proceed.

This isn't a race. Don't allow your ego to get ahead of your body's capacity for training and recuperation. One of the main reasons people discontinue working out is that they start out like gangbusters and before long wear themselves to a frazzle. More is definitely not better. You should ratchet up exercise quantity and frequency the same way your muscles grow and develop—a bit at a time.

I'd recommend that, before you begin the apprentice workouts, you read *all* of the next ten chapters so that you understand the overall thrust of the program.

Once you've read them through, go back to Week One and begin your seventy-day investment, one workout at a time. And make sure to do the motivation exercises in each chapter. Skipping them will only slow down your progress.

WEEK 1

This week I want you to decide exactly what your hopes and aspirations are for your flawlessness program. Don't be wishy-washy. Decide what you really want and go for it. All of your goals should be positive and filled with emotion. That is how you will get a concrete result.

Have you heard the saying "Be careful what you wish for—you might just get it"? When you set your mind to this task, I urge you to dream big. If you dream small you're likely to get small results. You should make sure your dream is close enough at hand to be rooted in reality, but sufficiently out of reach to give you something to push toward.

I'll talk a lot in this book about the mind-to-muscle link. Your mind fuels your muscles in many different ways. The most important at this stage are the nerve pathways, which will be built up and grow more efficient as you learn how to feel your muscles throughout the exercises.

Along with physical maintenance, machines need fuel, and many of you will start these ten weeks making dramatic changes in the fuel that you feed your machine. Don't think of this as a diet. Diet is really an acronym, you know. It means: Deprivation In Eating Till...till you can go right back to the way you used to eat, of course. The term suggests that there is some sort of magical stopping point—a point where the world stops spinning and you maintain with no effort. In fact, the contrary is the case. The nutritional plans in this program have been developed to instill lifetime habits.

JUST DO IT NOW

Procrastination is the death of every dream. If tomorrow is when you'll do it, then chances are you'll always put it off till tomorrow. Procrastination is usually rooted in fear. It is either a fear of failure or of success. "If I get a good body then I'll have to keep it and the work will never end."

Well, the work never does end. It's really a matter of finding passion in what you're doing. If you have passion for your workouts, nothing will keep you out of the gym.

TRAINING

The ten-week training program that I've developed for you contains exercises for all of the body parts described in the preceding chapters. Consult these sections as well as exercise instructions in this chapter if you have questions on exercise performance. In this Apprentice Program, you'll be training your whole body every other day. It could be Monday, Wednesday, Friday, or it could be Tuesday, Thursday, Saturday. Basically the structure should be that you follow one day of workout with one day of rest, and that after your week's third workout you take two days of rest.

The rest days will enable your body to recover from the stress placed on the muscles. Unless the muscles recover from one workout to the next, you will not make significant gains. I want you to plan an aerobic activity at least four times this first week. These workouts should be done on the days off from weights, so that you are stimulating your metabolism and alternating aerobic and anaerobic exercise days. As the weeks go on you'll increase the frequency and duration of your aerobic workouts, but for now let's take the first step and get started. Consult the preceding aerobics section for target heart rate information.

Consider the first two workouts this week as rehearsals. Go into the gym and go through each exercise, paying strict attention to the details of how they're properly executed. Don't worry about the weights you use. Instead, use very light weights (or maybe even a broomstick) and find the grooves. Learn where each movement's stretch point and contraction point is. Tense the muscles you're working as you go through these rehearsal workouts. Pay attention to how the muscle feels throughout the full range of motion. By the week's third workout you can begin to use weights that will allow you to do the recommended number of repetitions, but the exercises should still be done in super-strict style.

NUTRITION

As this program begins, your main nutritional concern should be achieving a clean, balanced diet. After that house is in order, we'll talk about what vitamins, minerals and aminos to take. You can walk into any health food store and see hundreds of products promising to help you do this, that or the other thing. But supplements are exactly what the term implies—substances that "supplement" the core eating program. They aren't meant to replace nutritious eating.

There are supplements that can bolster your nutritional needs. But taking supplements without a sound eating plan is like painting the outside of a house whose roof has caved in.

MOTIVATION

Sit in a quiet place where your body is relaxed. Your spine should be comfortably straight with your head upright, but without tension in the neck.

I want you to take a deep breath in through your nose. Hold the breath for half a second and then gently and evenly let it out through your mouth. As you breathe out, locate and relax all the tension spots in your body. Take between five and ten deep, cleansing breaths in this manner, each time relaxing tension spots as you exhale. Close your eyes after about the third breath. Once your body is fully relaxed, just breathe naturally and begin to imagine your flawless body. Picture your flawless body standing on top of a beautiful pedestal. The pedestal you imagine should be capable of revolving so that you can see your body from all angles. We won't use this revolving pedestal this week, but create it now anyway. Make it all real and vivid. See your goal body from head to toe just from the front. Examine it with care. Now intensify the image. Make it brighter or louder or stronger—whatever will "turn up the volume."

Remember to root this goal body to your structural reality. With intensity, imagine this for five minutes, and then let it go. Slowly open your eyes and make a short journal entry about the experience. Repeat this exercise at least four of the next seven days. Each time try to intensify the image.

Note about the weekly workout listings that follow: If you are in doubt about which body part is affected by the listed exercise, please consult exercise descriptions elsewhere in the book. Number ranges listed next to the exercise specify, first, the number of sets, and second, the repetition range.

APPRENTICE WEEK 1

Weights: Day #1...#3...#5

Flat Bench Presses	2	× 100	15–20
Low-Pulley Rows *reverse flies*	2	× 10	15–20
Barbell Press Behind Neck *military*	2	× 50	15–20
Barbell Curls	2	×	15–20
Tricep Push-downs *kickbacks*	2	×	15–20
Leg Presses *squats*	2	×	15–20
Lying Leg Curls	2	×	15–20
Leg-Press Raises *abs*	2	×	15–20
Crunches	2	×	15–20
Dumbbell Wrist Curls	2	×	15–20

Aerobics: Day #1...#2...#6...#7

AEROBICS

Select one aerobic exercise and do it at a moderate level (with your pulse at a 65 to 70 percent level) for fifteen to twenty minutes. If at any time you feel dizzy or overly out of breath, stop the exercise. I'd suggest beginning your aerobic workout program with stationary cycling or fast walking.

WEEK 2

At the beginning of each new week I want you to review what you've accomplished for the preceding seven days. For example, which body parts did you "feel" the best? Which ones were difficult? Were you able to follow your nutrition plan? Did you consistently visualize your flawless body? Did you read your contract to yourself twice each day? You should be keeping a day-by-day training journal and using one page at the end of each week to write a short review of your progress. Your notes can be elaborate or simple. I just want you to believe that if it's worth doing, it's worth writing down. These notes will come in very handy as you review how effective the ten weeks were for you.

During the next week you'll be getting a feel for those exercises that come easy as opposed to those that don't. All of us have our strengths and weaknesses. Strengths are usually easy to build on. Weaknesses, on the other hand, take some work. It's human nature to shy away from things that don't come easy.

There's no way for me to design these programs and tailor them perfectly to all the different body types and metabolisms of the people who will use them. This is where getting to know yourself becomes essential. Follow the programs to the letter, but adjust them to your own body by putting more intensity and effort into the areas where you need the most work. As I've said before, you need to fall in love with your weaknesses. This means using your passion, inspiration and hard work to turn a weak body part into a strong one. A body part becomes strong when it's visually in proportion with the rest of your body. I find an overdeveloped body part just as objectionable as an underdeveloped one.

When I first began training, my shoulders grew very quickly, but my biceps lagged behind. I would train shoulders with fire and enthusiasm and biceps with mediocre intensity. Then I figured out that this system wasn't working, that I was only going to build weird proportions this way. So I began to observe how I approached training shoulders—what I felt; what went through my mind; how I felt the muscle, etc.

I then began looking at and thinking about my biceps in a similar manner. Within no time my biceps gains accelerated. Also, I was that much more in touch with my shoulders because of all the observations I'd made. I saw the value of learning my own body and put it to practical use toward the physique I desired.

TRAINING

In the beginning, you need to understand that a weight workout is not a sprint. During these formative weeks you're trying to discover how your body works, not how fast you can get through your routine. The pace of your workouts will depend on your level of fitness and experience. First, though, let's get one thing straight: If you're in the gym working on this program and you want to see results by the end of ten weeks, you must not treat the gym as a social environment. If you're there mainly to talk to friends or get a date, this is not the program for you.

Concentration during and between exercises is going to be the key to your success in the gym. Between sets you should be focused on preparing yourself for whatever is coming next.

Your pace between exercises is going to depend on your breathing. Once you've finished a set on an exercise, you'll begin the next set when your breathing returns to a "hard" normal—in other words, not while you're panting, but not at your normal resting breath either. If you have nausea or dizziness or feel "out of it," sit down and really catch your breath fully before deciding whether to continue.

From one exercise to the next, rest just long enough to set up new equipment and to take a sip of water.

NUTRITION

Bad nutritional habits can be hard to break. There are people who eat to live and those who live to eat. I personally don't trust anyone who doesn't have a strong attachment to food, but I guess that's because I'm one of those "live to eat" types. Actually I'm joking about not trusting those "eat to live" folks. I've just always been envious of people who don't plan their next meal while eating the one in front of them. Earlier in my career I researched the way "eat to live" types look at food. What I found was that by doing this research I was thinking about food again, and it was this obsession that made all the difference. In fact an "eat to live" person would think I was crazy for doing the research in the first place. "Just eat," he'd say.

That's what he'd do, too: He'd eat what he wanted, only when he was hungry. He'd stop eating when he was satisfied and then wouldn't think of food again until hunger returned. Sounds pretty sick and twisted, huh? No, of course it doesn't. It just wasn't my style. In fact, it probably wouldn't work for most people on a bodybuilding program. Most of the people I help who are desperately trying to gain muscle and have tried everything fall into this "eat to live" category. It's hard for them to begin using a systematic meal pattern instead of an instinctive one. If you have a high metabolism, you *must* become an eating machine to gain weight. You must nudge your well-regulated metabolism off its plateau.

If losing body fat is your goal, you'll probably want to emulate the traits of an "eat to live" personality. But I'd suggest doing so using a systematic approach. As you replace junk food with clean food, learn to appreciate the positive difference. Your scheduled mealtimes will assure even blood sugar levels throughout the day and fewer of the cravings that come when blood sugar levels drop.

MOTIVATION

I want you to continue with the same visualization exercise you began last week. Quietly breathe yourself into relaxation and visualize your flawless body on a pedestal.

This week I want you to vividly and with full emotion feel that pedestal revolve so that you can see your flawless body from the front, sides and back. Experience what it feels like to be inside your flawless body for five or ten minutes for four out of the next seven days.

Continue to enter your observations in your journal.

APPRENTICE WEEK 2

Weights: Day #1...#3...#5

Incline Bench Presses	2	×	15–20
Front Pull-downs	2	×	15–20
Dumbbell Presses	2	×	15–20
Incline Dumbbell Curls	2	×	15–20
Lying Triceps Extensions	2	×	15–20
Back Squats	2	×	15–20
Lying Leg Curls	2	×	15–20
Standing Calf Raises	2	×	15–20
Lying Leg Raises	2	×	15–20
Barbell Wrist Curls	2	×	15–20

Aerobics: Day #2...#4...#6...#7

Do your aerobics in the same style as last week: at a 65 to 70 percent pulse rate for fifteen to twenty minutes.

WEEK 3

By now you should have a good sense of which of your body parts are stronger and which are weaker. This is the time, then, to take a long and serious look at what your body really looks like and to analyze what parts of the overall structure need the most work.

There's a very good reason why I've waited till the beginning of the third week to suggest this analysis. I wanted you to be totally familiar with what a biceps, lat or delt is. I wanted you to have felt each muscle work in the gym, moving the weights up and down.

Before you begin this week's workouts, find a place where you can use a full-length mirror in private. Take a hand-held mirror with you also. Strip off your clothes and stand in front of the mirror. In your journal, on an empty page, draw a line down the middle from top to bottom. On the top left side write "Strengths," and on the right "Weaknesses."

Now begin at the top of the body and work your way down the front, noting what you feel is visually strong or weak and writing it down. You should list only those physical features that you can change. (For example, you can't change your bone structure, height or foot size.) If you hate what you see, please don't use this as an opportunity to rake yourself over the coals and make yourself feel miserable. The key to this reality exercise is total honesty.

Now make this same analysis from both sides and, using the hand-held mirror, from the rear. Write it all down. Keep this page in your journal. You'll be going through this again and you need this for reference. Now, next to all aspects that you have listed as weaknesses, I want you to write a short goal sentence.

For example, if biceps are listed as a weakness, next to it you might write: "I'll learn to increase feeling and intensity on curls. I must increase my focus on this area." Make sure to state all of your goals in a positive way.

If the problem is with body fat or its distribution, write a sentence about how you'll solve this, too. This is not a long process. It should take you fifteen to twenty minutes at the most.

This self-inspection will help you to further root your expectations in reality.

TRAINING

You bring into this program a body that has a history. You have used—and probably abused—your body for the entire time you've been alive. The human machine was built to withstand a great deal of punishment. It was made to bend and not break under usual circumstances. But time and use bring with them wear and tear, whether you've been active or inactive.

Muscles, joints and tendons, like those rubber bands on a cold morning, become stiff and cranky. Low back, knees and elbows find ways to give new definition to pain. When it comes to that pain, the best medicine is prevention. If, however, an injury is already present, it becomes necessary to learn how to work around it to avoid further damage. This is one of the reasons for my almost obsessive emphasis on perfect exercise form. Ballistic (bouncing, throwing or jerking) movements treat your joints like a hammer would treat the hood of your car. The damage is right there—if not now, later.

There is, however, a major difference between right and wrong soreness. The wrong soreness is a pain that feels like something is ripping or snapping. The right soreness during and after a workout feels like muscles filling up with too much fluid and a burning sensation as blood and lactic acid flow into the muscle. Bodybuilders call this "the pump." As you probably already know from the past two weeks, the pump feels like having a bicycle pump attached to your muscles. Each repetition is like pushing the pump's handle up and down, filling up the muscles and making them feel tighter.

The right soreness after a workout is an indicator of a good training session. Usually muscle soreness from weight training sets in between one hour and two days after a workout. There should be a *slight* tenderness in the main part of the muscle. Self-massage and ice therapy can be extremely useful in helping to speed up the process of getting past this soreness. Use your fingers to massage the muscles you can reach and have someone assist you on your back muscles. Massage has been proven effective in muscle recovery.

The use of ice packs for five to fifteen minutes will substantially reduce muscle soreness by reducing the inflammation that takes place in the fibers after an intense training session.

NUTRITION

What is it that makes changing the way you eat so difficult? A large part of it is social conditioning. Let's assume that you're trying to lose body fat and have a history of eating a normal American diet. It's basically high-fat, high-sugar and low-fiber, but pretty tasty. Aren't the feelings you have from eating fatty beef sandwiches and deep-fried potatoes just mental associations you've derived from TV commercials telling you how you'll feel if you eat them? The problem carries over to cigarette ads. Advertisers have been able to take this foul, smelly, deadly and highly addictive drug and link people's associations with it to sexy models, fun in the sun, glamour or cartoon characters. You need to take back control from Madison Avenue.

Anytime you deprive your body of one of its necessities, you'll feel the pain. It's human nature to avoid pain and to find comfort at any cost. If an unhealthy style of eating has been comfortable for you, then you need to change your mind-set toward clean food. You've got to realize that the pain you're avoiding now if you're eating unhealthy is going to turn into larger pain in the long run.

You *must* find the pleasure in eating clean foods. Find the satisfaction of taking control of your machine and giving it the right fuel. Above all else, take your nutrition one day at a time. The reality of how you eat is right now, today. How you ate yesterday does not affect what you do today.

MOTIVATION

I want you to continue this week with the relaxation/visualization exercise you've already been working on. On four of the next seven days, breathe yourself down into a relaxed state. I want you to do this week's first visualization exercise immediately following your self-analysis in the mirror, as discussed earlier. This way you'll still have a fresh image of what your body really looks like in your mind. I want you to visualize yourself still on the revolving pedestal, but this time picture yourself in the body you have right now. Get a firm image of this first, then in your mind make the pedestal start to rotate, beginning at the front and working your way to your sides and back. As you look at your body from each angle, begin to change each body part the way you wanted it changed in your body analysis. It will be as if you're carving and perfecting a piece of sculpture. Go around your body a couple of times, making changes. Then spend a few minutes appreciating that flawless body you've just created.

It should look pretty similar to the one you've been imagining for the last two weeks, but perfect the image each time you work on it. Remember to alter only those physical traits that you'll be able to change through exercise and diet. An overriding purpose of this exercise is to begin to appreciate and respect the core physical elements you possess as you work toward positive change.

APPRENTICE WEEK 3

Weights: Day #1...#5

Flat Bench Presses	3	×	15–20
Low-Pulley Rowing	3	×	15–20
Barbell Presses Behind Neck	3	×	15–20
Barbell Curls	3	×	15–20
Triceps Pushdowns	3	×	15–20
Leg Presses	3	×	15–20
Lying Leg Curls	3	×	15–20
Standing Calf Raises	3	×	15–20
Crunches	3	×	15–20
Dumbbell Wrist Curls	3	×	15–20

Weights: Day #3

Inclines Bench Presses	3	×	15–20
Front Pull-downs	3	×	15–20
Dumbbell Presses	3	×	15–20
Incline Curls	3	×	15–20
Lying Triceps Extensions	3	×	15–20
Back Squats	3	×	15–20
Lying Leg Curls	3	×	15–20
Standing Calf Raises	3	×	15–20
Lying Leg Raises	3	×	15–20
Barbell Wrist Curls	3	×	15–20

Aerobics: Day #2...#4...#6...#7

Continue at 65 to 70 percent for fifteen to twenty minutes.

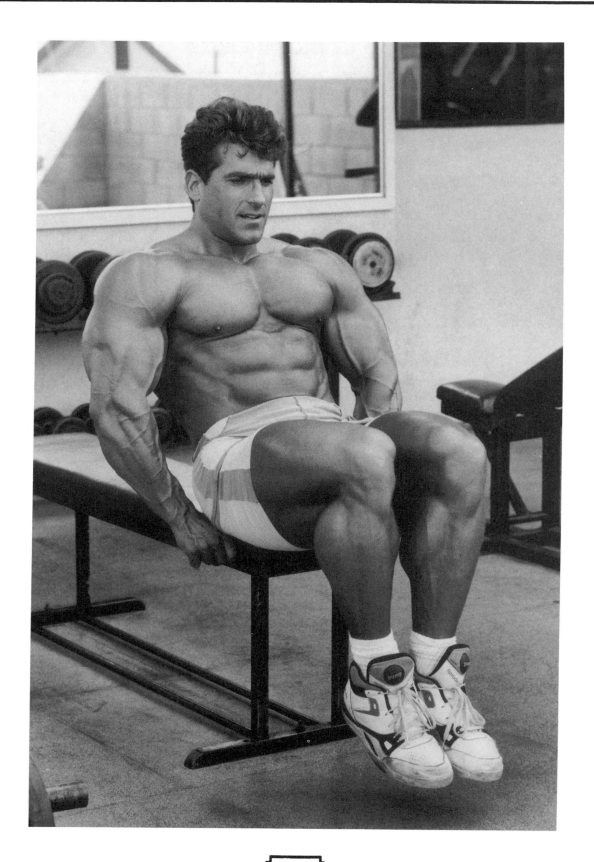

WEEK 4

This week I'd like to spend some time talking about goals. In my seminars I talk about how we are all setting goals on a daily basis. We are either setting goals that serve to improve our lives or ones that destroy our lives. People don't intend to set negative goals, but the mind is like a wild horse; if you don't control it, it will control you. Deep down, all of us want great things to happen in our lives—we're just never fully told how to go out and get them. We need to reprogram our lives by replacing destructive goals with ones that will enhance our health and self-esteem.

I seriously doubt if anyone would intentionally set a ten-week fitness goal that would cause him or herself harm. Yet many people behave as if their contract with themselves reads like this: "During the next ten weeks I'll do everything I can to destroy my health and looks to the greatest extent possible. I'll be completely inactive, get no exercise and eat a fatty, sugary diet filled with junk food. I'll smoke and drink to excess and won't take care of my outward appearance. Then in ten weeks I'll really be on my way to a new me."

This goal is not purposely set, yet it gets fulfilled by millions every day. You, on the other hand, have now felt what it's like to take charge of your goal-setting process. The contract you made with yourself was a major step. Doing the day-by-day work necessary to live up to your commitment is going to leave you successful and wanting more at the end of your program.

I heard a wonderful saying some time ago. I don't know who originally spoke the words, but they continue to give me hope.

"The past does not equal the future."

You can, at any point, no matter where you were yesterday, take charge of your life and develop a strategy for turning your dreams into realities.

TRAINING

What kind of strength increase should you be able to expect during the course of your program? This is a difficult question to answer with any degree of accuracy. There are so many factors involved that it makes it impossible for me to say that by Week 4 you should have increased your exercise poundages by X percent. First, you need to understand that there are many different ways to grow stronger from weight training besides just being able to lift more weight, especially in the apprentice stages.

Secondly, you must understand that "strength" in the general sense contains within it several different components that reside in individuals in varying degrees. There's power, endurance, stamina, etc. It should be obvious to you by now that if your only goal for the next several weeks is increasing the amount of weight you can throw around, this is the wrong program.

Should you expect to gain strength during the program, though? Of course. Aren't you growing stronger if, for example, the weights you use remain the same but you learn to do the exercise perfectly? Absolutely. Any of the following types of improvements will mean across-the-board progress:

1. **Exercise techniques are perfected.**
2. **A higher number of repetitions are achieved with the same amount of weight.**
3. **Less rest time is necessary between sets.**
4. **While maintaining good form and the same repetition range, the weight is increased.**

Remember also that you're trying to sculpt your body with the exercises and weights you're using. The *amount* of weight being used is irrelevant as long as the set is well executed and is carried out to positive failure.

If I had my way, there'd be no numbers on the dumbbells and barbells in gyms. The average trainer places too much importance on the amount of weight used and too little on what it's being used for. If there weren't any numbers on the weights, you'd search more for the dumbbell or barbell that worked best. Yes, you want to grow stronger, but not at the sacrifice of progressing toward a flawless body.

NUTRITION

What do you do if you break your diet for a day? Let's say you become overwhelmed and go on a major binge, causing your weight to go up a couple of pounds. Or let's say you're trying to gain weight, have a hard time eating in the first place and completely blow off eating for a whole day, and as a result your weight drops a couple of pounds. In either case you should just concede that you lack the requisite willpower and give up, right? Wrong! You should pick yourself up, take stock of the goals you want your nutrition to achieve and resume the quest. Begin today. Let yesterday be a lesson in how painful breaking your plan can be. The pain of guilt and setback can be used to your advantage in sticking to your goals. When you failed to follow your nutrition plan you were, in some way, trying to make yourself feel good. The good feeling was temporary and the net result was actually feeling bad. Always try to keep in mind that your nutrition plan will make you feel great in the long run and that momentary gratification is not an equal trade-off for long-term happiness.

MOTIVATION

By now you should be well practiced at imagining your flawless body while doing your visualization exercises.

This week I want you to put that imaginary body into action while in the relaxed state. Once you've breathed yourself into relaxation, I want you to imagine your flawless body on the revolving pedestal. As the pedestal revolves, see your body from the front, back and side.

Then look away from your body to an imaginary wall next to the pedestal. On that wall I want you to create a door; make it as elaborate or simple as you like. It should be personal, vivid and inviting. It is the doorway to your dreams. Now look back to your body up on the pedestal, realizing that the door is still there even as you look away. Watch as you step down off the pedestal and move toward the doorway.

Reach out and open the door. On the other side is a place that is safe and good. It is a place where you have achieved your goals.

Remember in the Introduction how I had you picture yourself having achieved your wildest dream? I want you to do that again now, but before you walk through your door, I want you to say these words inside your head: "I control the doorway to my success." As soon as you say those words walk through the door.

On the other side is the world where you've achieved your dreams. Walk into that world and live inside your flawless body within that environment. A few minutes later, slowly bring yourself back into your present world. Sit and just breathe deeply for a couple of minutes, and remind yourself before you rush off to life again, "I control the doorway to my success."

APPRENTICE WEEK 4

Weights: Day #1 ... #5

Incline Bench Presses	3	×	15–20
Front Pull-downs	3	×	15–20
Dumbbell Presses	3	×	15–20
Incline Curls	3	×	15–20
Lying Triceps Extensions	3	×	15–20
Back Squats	3	×	15–20
Lying Leg Curls	3	×	15–20
Standing Calf Raises	3	×	15–20
Lying Leg Raises	3	×	15–20
Barbell Wrist Curls	3	×	15–20

Weights: Day #3

Flat Bench Presses	3	×	15–20
Low-Pulley Rowing	3	×	15–20
Barbell Presses Behind Neck	3	×	15–20
Barbell Curls	3	×	15–20
Triceps Push-downs	3	×	15–20
Leg Presses	3	×	15–20

Lying Leg Curls	3	×	15–20
Leg-Press Raises	3	×	15–20
Crunches	3	×	15–20
Dumbbell Wrist Curls	3	×	15–20

Aerobics: Day #2...#4...#6...#7

Increase your intensity to a pulse range of 70 to 75 percent and go for twenty minutes each session. If this is too intense, decrease either your pulse rate (to 65 percent) or your time (to fifteen minutes).

SELF-EVALUATION PRIOR TO WEEK 5

Before you begin your fifth week, I want you to evaluate your progress. The point of this evaluation is to determine whether to continue on the Apprentice Program or to advance to the beginning of the next level. I want you to take this evaluation very seriously and to be honest with yourself.

You aren't going to do yourself any good if you move to a more intense level before your body has had a chance to adapt to its present workload.

If you look ahead at the remaining weeks of the Apprentice Program, you'll see that even the apprentice workouts will be increasing in volume and exercise variety; consider this also during your evaluation. In fact, there are several factors I want you to consider.

The first is what level of training experience you had when you started the program. If you were an absolute beginner, then chances are great that if I were teaching you in person I'd have you continue with the Apprentice Program. If you were coming back to training after a long layoff and the workouts were too easy, then I'd probably move you to the next level. And I want you to consider these other factors when making your decision:

1. **How well has my body adapted to this level?**
2. **How well are my muscles recovering after each workout?**

3. **Am I comfortable enough with my current knowledge to move on or should I stay and gain experience?**
4. **Since journeyman workouts involve a greater time commitment, can I realistically make this investment?**
5. **Are the workouts too hard or too easy for me?**
6. **If they're too easy, am I doing everything possible to work at a high intensity level?**

After answering these questions, you should be able to make an intelligent decision about your next move. About 75 percent of the time, I recommend to the people I work with that they stay with and complete the program they've begun. This evaluation is here for those 25 percent of you who may feel held back at this level.

If you decide to move up one level, I'd like you to first read and absorb all the introductions to the remaining Apprentice weeks. They're filled with knowledge that will help guide your way. Then, I'd like for you to go to the first week of the Journeyman Program and begin your next six weeks from there, moving from Week 1 through Week 6. Week Six will be the conclusion of your ten-week program. Stick with the same nutrition program you're now using.

If you've decided to stay in this program, well...that's great. We have a lot more ground to cover. As I said before, your workouts are going to increase in volume and become a bit more sophisticated. Please continue to read and absorb. Get into the gym; make your exercises more perfect than ever; eat right and do your visualization exercises.

Don't be afraid to peek ahead at the more advanced section. It's also filled with tips that you'll be using in the future if you decide to continue with your flawlessness goals.

WEEK 5

As I'm sure you've already discovered, when it comes to weight training and sound nutrition, there are no miracles. That's because we generally regard miracles as shortcuts. There are only so many shortcuts you can take in a fitness program before diminishing returns set in.

You've seen during the past month that your program will only give you what you are willing to give it. If you don't go into the gym, your body will know it. If you skip your visualization exercises and then wonder why you're not motivated, you're getting out what you put in.

You already know the benefits of putting forth the physical and mental effort toward attaining your goal. At the end of this week you'll be halfway to reaching that goal. At the end of the ten weeks you might want to ask yourself which was more important: reaching the goal, or the work and planning that went into achieving it?

We've all heard the saying that "Life is a journey, not a destination." I'm hoping that as you invest more of your time and energy into your health and self-esteem, this clichéd saying will take on real meaning. It's my hope that as the weeks go by, training and good nutrition will become as second nature to you as brushing your teeth.

TRAINING

For many apprentices, the most difficult aspect of training to grasp is the concept of intensity. Just what is intensity as it relates to your workout program?

I think of intensity as the exertion of tremendous concentration and/or power. In weight training, this means focusing full attention on the exercise you're performing and doing that exercise with full physical power. Intensity on a set carried to positive failure would involve using perfect exercise form but still putting tremendous will and drive behind each repetition. The line you must be careful not to cross is getting so "into" a set that you begin to throw the weight around, thinking that it will increase the intensity.

"Positive failure" is a concept that I'd like to expand on in this section. In the workouts you've been following, your exercises have generally been in the range of fifteen to twenty repetitions. When you're doing the exercise, does that mean you stop at twenty repetitions even if you know you could continue in good form for a couple more? No. You should continue until you can do no more repetitions while still maintaining exercise perfection. On the next set you should adjust the weight so that positive failure is more likely to happen inside the target repetition range.

NUTRITION

Are you bored with your diet? Can't wait for the ten weeks to be over so that you can go back to eating "normal"?

Set those feelings aside for a minute and let's talk about long-range nutrition goals. During these ten weeks, you're trying to make the greatest amount of change in the shortest time possible. So you have something to work toward. What I hope you learn during this time period is that you should always be looking toward an outcome. If you don't plan it, then it won't be the outcome you desire. I'd like for you to take the long-range view with nutrition. Your eating now should be more than just getting from point A to point B. It should be the beginning of new and healthy habits that can serve you. It may sound corny, but you must make food your servant, not be its slave. If you work in the right direction, the food you eat will help you stay healthy and look great. It's up to you.

I can tell you this, though: Yo-yo dieting does not work. Every time you get lean, then fat, lean and fat, you increase your body's ability to efficiently store fat. You also dramatically increase your risk of a number of ailments, from heart disease to diabetes—not to mention the low self-esteem you undoubtedly feel during your free-time.

You need the right fuel to make the machine go the distance in style.

MOTIVATION

This week I want you to continue with your visualization exercise from last week. Remember to strive to make your imagination stronger, brighter and clearer each time you practice. Stick it out.... these exercises are having an effect.

During this ten-week program, I want you to reach for more than just improved physical appearance and health; I want you to work toward changing and improving the way you look at your body and yourself. Part of that is going to involve affirming a new belief system.

Let's therefore take the visualization exercises a step further now. I want you to write down affirmations that you feel will contribute to your goals.

Get ten 3×5 cards. On each card I want you to write one positive affirmation that relates to your goals. Make each one very positive and word it so that you've already accomplished the goal. For example: "I follow my nutrition plan with dedication and discipline," or "I do everything in my power to accomplish my flawlessness program goals."

Cover all aspects of your program: training, aerobics, nutrition and motivation. After you've filled out all ten cards, put a rubber band around them and carry them with you in your pocket at all times.

At least twice a day I want you to pull out your affirmation cards and read each one. As you do, feel the full impact and emotion of having this goal under complete control. Spend five or ten seconds feeling each affirmation. The whole process will take less than two minutes, but will be extraordinarily motivating. Root your affirmations in reality and only strive to change that which you can change.

APPRENTICE WEEK 5

Weights: Day #1 . . . #5

Flat Bench Presses	2	×	15–20
Incline Dumbbell Flyes	2	×	12–15
Front Pull-downs	2	×	12–15
Low-Pulley Rows	2	×	15–20
Dumbbell Presses	2	×	15–20
Dumbbell Side Raises	2	×	12–15
Barbell Curls	4	×	12–15
Push-downs	4	×	15–20
Leg Presses	2	×	15–20
Extensions	2	×	12–15
Lying Leg Curls	3	×	12–15
Hyperextensions	2	×	15–20
Leg-Press Raises	4	×	15–20
Crunches	2	×	15–20
Lying Leg Raises	2	×	15–20
Dumbbell Wrist Curls	3	×	15–20

Weights: Day #3

Incline Bench Presses	2	×	12–15
Flat Dumbbell Flyes	2	×	15–20
Rear Pull-downs	2	×	15–20
Low-Pulley Rows	2	×	15–20
Barbell Presses Behind Neck	2	×	12–15
Bent-over Side Raises	2	×	15–20
Incline Curls	4	×	15–20
Lying French Presses	4	×	15–20
Extensions	2	×	15–20
Back Squats	2	×	12–15
Lying Leg Curls	3	×	15–20
Hyperextensions	2	×	12–15
Standing Calf Raises	2	×	15–20
Seated Calf Raises	2	×	15–20
Lying Leg Raises	2	×	12–15
Scissors	2	×	12–15
Barbell Wrist Curls	3	×	12–15

Aerobics: Day #2 . . . #4 . . . #6 . . . #7

Keep your pulse rate in the range of 70 to 75 percent and increase the duration to twenty to twenty-five minutes each session.

WEEK 6

Now that you're into the last half of this program, there are things that you can do to keep enthusiastically moving forward and making progress.

Earlier I defined enthusiasm as a passionate interest in doing the work that will accomplish a desired goal. "Passionate interest" is the key. That type of interest can be very difficult to maintain on a long-term basis. People usually picture enthusiasm as a lot of jumping up and down and rah-rah cheerleading. Enthusiastically pursuing a goal doesn't always have to involve an adrenaline rush, though. Your levels of motivation will fluctuate over the course of time. It's far more important to keep moving in the desired direction. You should take advantage of highly motivated times, but keep pushing on when motivation is lagging. Just pushing on will bolster motivation by moving you closer to your goal and farther away from those things you don't like about yourself.

TRAINING

I'm sure that by now you've had days in the gym when the weights seemed to be wearing wings and almost lifted themselves, and that there were days when the exact same poundage felt ten times heavier. This was your body going through its natural up-and-down cycles.

Don't be discouraged on those days that seem a bit "off." If your muscles aren't feeling especially strong, then redouble your focus on the *feel* of the muscle. Believe me, you'll have a stronger day again. It's just a natural rhythm. Because you're working on a relatively short program and want maximum results, it's essential to do the workout whether you feel like it or not (unless, of course, you're ill or injured). If you head to the gym and your mind's just not into it, go in anyway. Don't worry if you're not driven to have your best workout of the week, just start doing the exercises and focus on what you're doing. Chances are that by the time you're a quarter of the way

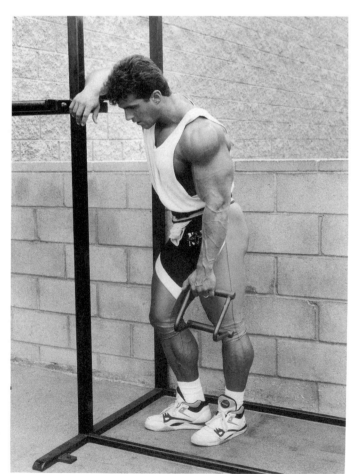

When you sense that you're having an "off day," redouble your focus.

through, you'll be having a good training session. And you'll find it hard to remember that you ever wanted to turn around, go home and lay in front of the tube.

Remember that motivation feeds on itself in a circular cycle. Doing the work makes you want to do more work. Go in and feel your muscles work. The rewards will be obvious.

NUTRITION

I want you to add something slightly esoteric to your nutrition plan that will benefit your recuperation and, in turn, your progress. You should follow the advice I'm about to give no matter which nutrition program you are currently using.

Your muscles function with glycogen as a primary fuel source. During the course of a weight-training session, you'll burn quite a bit of glycogen that has been stored in the muscle. A major portion of muscle recuperation relies on replacing that burned glycogen as quickly as possible after the workout.

Ideally your glycogen resupply will come from broken-down carbohydrates. Carbs represent the most efficient source of muscle glycogen and are the perfect choice for its postworkout replacement. Immediately after the workout is your system's most receptive time for glycogen replacement. Eating carbs at that time raises glycogen replacement to a level between four and ten times greater than if you waited even forty-five minutes to eat the same food.

So I want you to begin to take one source of complex carbohydrate to the gym with you (or if you train at home, to have it ready in the kitchen). Immediately after your workout I want you to consume this food. This shouldn't be a big meal; it should be just enough to replace your exhausted glycogen stores, but not enough to upset your stomach. Your food choices could be:

1. **A large apple**
2. **A large, plain baked potato**
3. **A cup of rice**
4. **A cup of oatmeal**
5. **A complex-carbohydrate drink mixed with water**

Do not consume any protein source at this time—the protein will interfere with glycogen replenishment. Don't fix a protein drink or a protein/carb drink and think that the results will be the same—they won't.

About half an hour to an hour later, you can eat your normal meal and continue with your regular plan.

MOTIVATION

Once again, find your quiet place. Breathe yourself down into a relaxed state; your mind and body should be fully relaxed. Using the same exercise you have been doing, watch your flawless body as the pedestal makes one full revolution. Watch yourself step down and walk toward the doorway. Before opening the door and going inside, see yourself saying, "I control the doorway to my success."

Once you're on the other side of the door, see yourself, still in your flawless body, dressed in workout clothes and in the gym where you train. Before you begin this visualization exercise I want you to pick the three or four weight exercises that you find most difficult. Now spend the next several minutes watching your flawless body do these exercises. Watch yourself use perfect form. Make your imaginary self both controlled and full of energy. Picture the sets being performed with maximum intensity. Do all the repetitions in your mind. Imagine your flawless self feeling the burn in the muscles and the intense satisfaction of a perfect set. Do at least one full set for all the exercises. When you are finished go back to the door and tell yourself, "I control the doorway to my success." Go through and then slowly bring yourself back to a wide-awake state.

Remember, really feel all those emotions; they'll carry over to boost your enthusiasm when you actually do walk into the gym. During the next weeks, use this technique on any area of your program that you need to physically strengthen. Picture yourself in your flawless body doing the activity perfectly and with motivation. Continue, at least twice a day, reading and feeling your affirmation cards. If you haven't begun, start now. Even if it sounds strange to you, do it. It works.

APPRENTICE WEEK 6

Weights: Day #1 ... #5

Incline Bench Presses	2	×	12–15
Flat Dumbbell Flyes	2	×	15–20
Rear Pull-downs	2	×	15–20
Low-Pulley Rows	2	×	12–15
Barbell Presses Behind Neck	2	×	12–15
Bent-over Side Raises	2	×	15–20
Incline Curls	4	×	15–20
Lying French Presses	4	×	15–20
Leg Extensions	2	×	15–20
Back Squats	2	×	12–15
Lying Leg Curls	3	×	15–20
Hyperextensions	2	×	12–15
Standing Calf Raises	2	×	15–20
Seated Calf Raises	2	×	15–20
Hanging Leg Raises	2	×	12–15
Scissors	2	×	12–15
Barbell Wrist Curls	3	×	12–15

Weights: Day #3

Flat Bench Presses	2	×	15–20
Incline Dumbbell Flyes	2	×	12–15
Front Pull-downs	2	×	12–15
Low-Pulley Rows	2	×	15–20
Dumbbell Presses	2	×	15–20
Dumbbell Side Raises	2	×	12–15
Barbell Curls	4	×	12–15
Push-downs	4	×	15–20
Leg Presses	2	×	15–20
Leg Extensions	2	×	12–15
Lying Leg Curls	3	×	12–15
Hyperextensions	2	×	15–20
Leg-Press Raises	4	×	15–20
Crunches	2	×	15–20
Lying Leg Raises	2	×	15–20
Dumbbell Wrist Curls	3	×	15–20

Aerobics: Day #2 ... #4 ... #6 ... #7

Continue working for twenty to twenty-five minutes in the pulse range of 70 to 75%. Try to vary your exercise as much as possible. Don't just get stuck using the bike; try the stair machine and walking, too.

WEEK 7

> **"Never give in. Never. Never. Never. Never."**
>
> —Winston Churchill

Keep pushing. Your goal is in sight. Whatever you do, don't give up. You've invested a lot of time and energy into moving toward your flawless body.

There is one thing I want you to prove to yourself during this program that goes beyond getting your body and health in shape. I'm talking about proving to yourself that you can do it. Don't underestimate the power of self-belief in pushing through and getting the job done.

Wisely used, persistence will always pay off. You might be going along, thinking that you're making no progress at all but pushing ahead anyway. Suddenly you turn a corner and there you are, standing face to face with a successfully realized goal. Was it a miracle? Well, there was no trick involved, but there was perhaps a bit of magic—the magic that happens when you put your nose to the grindstone day after day and results accumulate and expand.

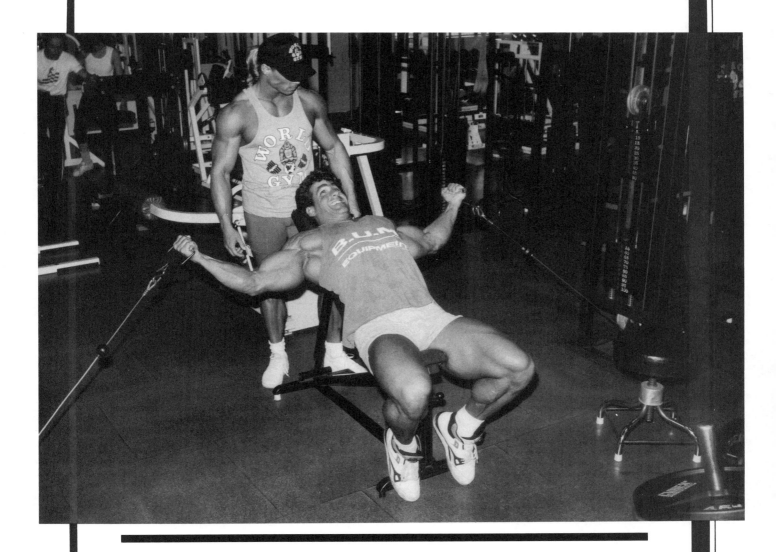

TRAINING

Everyone has stubborn body parts. In the beginning of my career my stubborn body part was my chest. I thought that I was doing everything that I could to build my chest muscles. I was ready to abandon that body part as just being inferior to the rest of my physique, but I didn't. Instead, I dug in. I became determined to become more stubborn than the muscle could ever be. In the end, I won. I persisted in seeking out new ways to bring development to my lagging pecs. I investigated the muscle's physiology and structure. I tried to discover where all that work I thought I was doing for my chest was really going. I became obsessed with correct alignment and exercise perfection. My chest responded, and to this day I can't do one repetition on a chest exercise without fully sinking myself into the feeling. If I don't feel it, then I know I'm cheating myself.

The tendency most people have is to shy away from weaker body parts. They work what grows easily, and the imbalance between strength and weakness grows greater. If you invest your greatest effort in your weakest body parts, before you know it you'll have created a strength. Be stubbornly persistent in your pursuit of a balanced physique.

NUTRITION

You will be tempted every day, from every conceivable source, to stray away from your clean-eating plan. Television ads; magazine ads; fast-food restaurants along the road; well-intentioned but misguided friends and relatives. Whatever the source of trouble might happen to be, stay on track.

When I'm having heavy-duty cravings, even walking into the supermarket can be a nightmare. I've learned to solve the problem, at least partially, by only going down aisles that have exactly what I need. There are no fresh vegetables in the cookie aisle. Fresh fish isn't usually kept by bulk bins of candy. Make a list and plan your route. Most of what you'll need—vegetables, fruits, meat and eggs—will be stocked around the perimeter of the store. You will usually have to go down aisles for rice, oatmeal, spices...that kind of stuff. Do yourself two favors in advance of shopping:

1. **Go to the store after a meal, not while you're hungry.**
2. **Get in and get out. Don't drool over the ingredients in cake mixes; you'll be setting yourself up to undermine your goal. You're getting closer every day. You have to keep pushing to make it work.**

MOTIVATION

Continue with your visualization exercises. Really focus on these exercises on days when your enthusiasm isn't as high as you would like. Make the images bright, focused and clear.

Continue to read and feel your affirmation cards at least twice a day.

One of the methods that I use to mentally make it through a set on an exercise is to break up my repetition counting in different ways. For example, let's say I'm trying to do twenty reps on a set. I might do something like count backward as I do the reps. The first one would be 20, the second 19, and so on till I get to 1. Don't ask me why this works better for me than counting from 1 to 20, because I can't give you a scientific answer. (Perhaps it's that this makes it more like a countdown for a rocket blast-off, so I feel the intensity build more.)

You can also break the set up into number blocks, like groupings of five reps. You do the set the same way, except you just count 1 through 5, 1 through 5, until the set is finished. For me, this makes the set seem shorter, and four groupings of five reps feels like less work than twenty reps. I just try to be creative to keep my mind focused on the set and to keep boredom from creeping in.

APPRENTICE WEEK 7

Weights: Day #1...#5

Flat Bench Presses	2	×	15–20
Incline Dumbbell Flyes	2	×	12–15
Front Pull-downs	2	×	12–15
Low-Pulley Rows	2	×	15–20
Dumbbell Presses	2	×	15–20
Dumbbell Side Raises	2	×	12–15
Barbell Curls	4	×	12–15
Push-downs	4	×	15–20
Leg Presses	2	×	15–20
Leg Extensions	2	×	12–15
Lying Leg Curls	3	×	12–15
Hyperextensions	2	×	15–20
Leg-Press Raises	4	×	15–20
Crunches	2	×	15–20
Lying Leg Raises	2	×	15–20
Dumbbell Wrist Curls	3	×	15–20

Weights: Day #3

Incline Bench Presses	2	×	12–15
Flat Dumbbell Flyes	2	×	15–20
Rear Pulldowns	2	×	15–20
Low-Pulley Rows	2	×	12–15
Barbell Presses Behind Neck	2	×	12–15
Bent-over Side Raises	2	×	15–20
Incline Curls	4	×	15–20
Lying French Presses	4	×	15–20
Leg Extensions	2	×	15–20
Back Squats	2	×	12–15
Lying Leg Curls	3	×	15–20
Hyperextensions	2	×	12–15
Standing Calf Raises	2	×	15–20
Seated Calf Raises	2	×	15–20
Lying Leg Raises	2	×	12–15
Scissors	2	×	12–15
Barbell Wrist Curls	3	×	12–15

Aerobics: Day #2 ... #6

Continue doing twenty to twenty-five minutes in the pulse range of 70 to 75 percent.

Aerobics: Day #4 ... #7

Move your duration up to twenty-five to thirty minutes and try to keep your pulse around 75 percent.

WEEK 8

It's entirely possible to be hard and gentle on yourself at the same time. It's a matter of knowing when each is appropriate and exercising discipline and patience as they're needed.

Most people give up on training and/or good nutrition because they're too hard on themselves. There are lots of ways for you to be too hard on yourself; most revolve around impatience. For example, take the person who wants a great body *now* and throws himself into a workout far above his needs or experience level. He either gets so sore that he never goes back to the gym, or overtrains so badly that no progress can be made and he quits in frustration.

Or how about the person who begins a program and can't stick with it out of what appears to be laziness. Isn't he really just returning to what is familiar and comfortable? If he were persistent and patient, he'd see old, destructive habits replaced by new, healthy ones.

New, healthier habits need to gather steam and be attached in our minds to good feelings to push the old ones out of the way. Your perspective on your life can change in a second, but becoming "addicted" will always take time and patience.

Keep pushing. The light is in sight at the end of the tunnel.

TRAINING

All sorts of negative things will happen when you get impatient in your workouts, injury and overtraining being the two most common.

Overtraining means that you are doing more work in the gym than your body, at its current experience level, has the ability to recover from. Let's say you're not satisfied to only do X number of sets on an exercise and decide to double the number. If your body isn't ready for the workload, it will respond by not fully recovering for the next workout. It's sort of like paying your bills with a credit card. You're putting your body into recovery debt, and the effects "gather interest" quickly. Muscle recuperation is as essential to your progress as the exercises themselves. More is definitely not always better.

Injuries happen when you aren't focusing on exercise form and the feel of the muscle. Some people try to increase poundages before the body and system are ready and dramatically sacrifice form for ego. Stick to your program and to exercise perfection. Your results will be consistent and long-term.

NUTRITION

Every one of us knows at least one person who is on the diet roller coaster; perhaps, before you started this program, you were on it yourself.

The bookstores are filled with thousands of up-to-the-minute, "miracle," "wonder" diet books. We are a culture obsessed with quick visual fixes for long-term internal abuses. Every time you go on a miracle diet (you know—"Celebrity loses 300 pounds on a buttered popcorn, pine needle tea and strawberry pop-tart diet"), you are opting for the gimmicky solution. Which is *no* solution."

That's why the nutrition plan you've been following is designed around balanced, clean nutrition instead of gimmick foods. Look, it would be easy for me to write a gimmick diet book—*Mr. Universe's Maple Syrup Diet for Rippling Abdominals*—and it would probably make a fortune. But it would only feed, like a shark, off people's desires for painless change.

In the Appendix, you will see differences among the programs based on individual goals, metabolisms and body types, but they all have one element in common—balance. They also contribute to the goal of helping you make positive changes in your eating habits, so that you'll not only feel better, but feel better about yourself.

You know...no more yo-yo.

MOTIVATION

Continue with your visualization exercises. Really focus on these exercises on days when your enthusiasm isn't as high as you'd like.

This week, change your affirmation cards. Create ten to twelve brand-new positive cards for yourself. Make them personal and emotional and write them as if the goal is already accomplished. For example, "I follow my positive nutrition plan with great enthusiasm. I look forward to each meal." Keep using the cards at least twice a day and fully feel the emotion as you read each one. If you use them daily, I can guarantee that you'll be charged up to go out and fulfill that goal. You'll be replacing self-defeating thought patterns with enriching ones.

Remember, either you control your mind or it controls you. If you aren't controlling the input into your mind, all kinds of outside influences are willing to do it for you.

APPRENTICE WEEK 8

Weights: Day #1...#5

Incline Bench Presses	2	×	15–20
Incline Dumbbell Flyes	2	×	12–15
Flat Dumbbell Flyes	2	×	12–15
Front Pull-downs	2	×	15–20
Rear Pull-downs	2	×	12–15
Low-Pulley Rows	2	×	12–15
Barbell Presses Behind Neck	2	×	15–20
Bent-over Side Raises	2	×	15–20
Barbell Curls	4	×	15–20
Push-downs	3	×	12–15
Lying French Presses	3	×	12–15
Leg Presses	2	×	15–20
Leg Extensions	2	×	12–15
Lying Leg Curls	3	×	15–20
Hyperextensions	2	×	12–15
Standing Calf Raises	4	×	12–15
Crunches	2	×	15–20
Lying Leg Raises	2	×	15–20
Dumbbell Wrist Curls	3	×	15–20

Weights: Day #3

Flat Bench Presses	2	×	12–15
Incline Bench Presses	2	×	12–15
Low-Pulley Row	2	×	15–20
Rear Pull-downs	2	×	15–20
Dumbbell Presses	2	×	12–15
Dumbbell Side Raises	2	×	12–15
Bent-over Side Raises	2	×	12–15
Incline Dumbbell Curls	3	×	12–15
Barbell Curls	3	×	12–15
Push-downs	4	×	15–20
Leg Extensions	2	×	15–20
Leg Presses	2	×	12–15
Lying Leg Curls	3	×	12–15
Hyperextensions	2	×	15–20
Leg-Press Raises	3	×	15–20
Seated Calf Raises	3	×	12–15
Lying Leg Raises	2	×	15–20
Scissors	2	×	12–15
Barbell Wrist Curls	4	×	12–15

Aerobics

Continue using the same duration and intensity pattern as last week.

WEEK 9

Two more weeks to go. Your goal is right there in front of you.

How has the experience of the past eight weeks been for you? Have you been enjoying your adventure? Or has it been a chore and a drag?

I hope it has been a great adventure, during which you've learned tons about how your body works. Let's take a moment to review the key knowledge you've accumulated so far:

1. Training with weights is much more than just swinging weights around. In order to be successful and avoid injury, you must learn to feel the muscles being focused on.

2. Perfect exercise form is more important to your progress than lifting the heaviest weight you can pick up.

3. The combination of weight training, aerobics, good nutrition and motivational exercises is synergistic—the outcome from the combination far exceeds the result that would be experienced if any of the elements were left out.

4. Dietary supplements cannot make up for a poor diet. You must first develop a clean, balanced eating strategy that suits your goals and metabolism. Follow it diligently before even considering adding supplementation.

5. If you break your workout or nutrition plan, you should get right back on track. You shouldn't beat yourself up over it. Just pick up where you left off and move on.

6. There are several different ways to grow stronger in your workouts. Increasing the amount of weight used is only one.

7. All of your goals for a flawless body should be rooted in the reality of your body structure and your ability to invest time and effort.

8. You've learned how to visualize your flawless body in action. That vision is the drawing board on which you can sketch further images of success.

9. "Just do it now" is a personal rallying cry that will get you to push forward when you feel like doing anything else in the world rather than training and eating clean.

10. Through perfecting your exercise form, you've learned the difference between appropriate pain, such as the burn in the muscle, and injurious pain.

11. Positive affirmation cards can plant emotional success messages. The process has begun to replace negative body images with high self-esteem.

12. You know now that you can do it. You have the ability to physically control your body through exercise and nutrition.

13. Rest and recuperation are as essential to your gains as the exercise itself.

14. Yo-yo, crash dieting *never* works.

15. You've learned to use positive failure as a guideline for when a set is complete. You've used focus and concentration to give your fullest power to each set.

It's my hope that you have learned these things and much more. This week I want you to continue with great passion, doing your training, nutrition, visualization and affirmation cards.

Two weeks to go. Use them to their fullest.

TRAINING

Whenever you train in a gym where lots of people work out, you're going to see some pretty strange training techniques. Now, that doesn't mean that you can't learn by watching others work out. I'd say, though, that most of what you should learn from these observations is how *not* to train.

Most people, unless they've worked with someone legitimately knowledge-able about exercise techniques, train with extraordinarily sloppy form. Why is that? I think it's because of the "loner" aspect of working out. There's no team effort, and quality coaching is sadly lacking; it's every person for himself. Most teaching materials on the subject cover stretches, sets and rows, with little or no emphasis on perfect form. As you know, I strongly feel that this thinking is backward.

My point is this: Stick to your exercise-perfection "guns"; focus in on your exercises and make them work for you. If you see someone doing an exercise that looks interesting, analyze it by observing what body part(s) it's intended to work. Then examine its mechanics in terms of what you already know about exercises for that body part. Refer back to "How the Muscles Work" to review the right grooves and mechanical actions for the muscle. No matter what exercise you're doing, always find the right stretch and contraction first. Then find the pathway that the weight will travel between the two. You now have the experience to know when something feels right and what part of the body it will work.

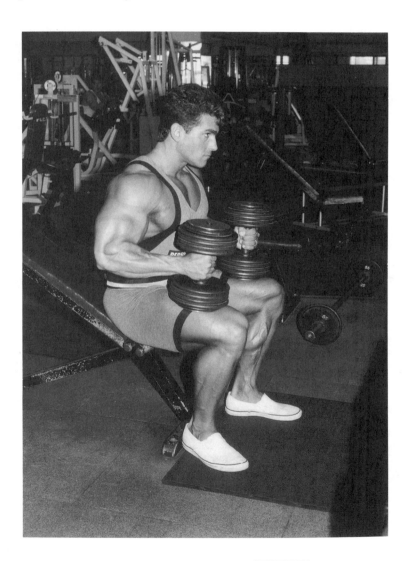

NUTRITION

What should you do when you eat out in a restaurant? The first thing to look for is a place that has a varied menu so you have different foods to choose from. Most fast-food chains are at least trying to make adjustments to fit Americans' changing eating habits. But, I don't care if french fries are prepared in lard or canola oil, either way, they're pure fat, no matter what advertisers try to tell you. In almost every case, you'll be breaking your nutrition plan by eating at a fast-food place.

There are good things happening at some of the chain coffee shops, though. Many now have entrees of skinless chicken breast or broiled fish. Many have baked potatoes available at any time of the day.

Always look for the lowest-fat meats. Ask for your baked potatoes dry (without butter or sour cream) and your vegetables plain-steamed. Salads should be eaten with either diet dressing or lemon and vinegar. Regular salad dressing will add tons of fat-filled calories to an innocent-looking plate of greens. You might as well have chocolate cake.

Ask your server to have your food prepared with no butter, oil or salt. Tell him or her that it's very important, and if it's not right, send it back. Also, don't fool yourself into believing a food is fat-free if it tastes richer than when you make it clean at home. When you find restaurants that accommodate your needs, stick with them.

MOTIVATION

It's time to go back in front of that full-length mirror to make a truthful and thorough physical analysis. Just as you did in Week 3, draw a line down the middle of a blank page in your journal, labeling the top of one side "Strengths" and the other side "Weaknesses."

Take off all of your clothes and analyze your body—front, side and rear, top to bottom. You're now fully familiar with all the body parts. You know what your strengths and weaknesses are in the gym. How do your strongest exercises correspond to your best body parts? How do your weakest exercises correspond with your weakest body parts? Write all of this down. Cover everything. Flip back to your first analysis and compare your notes. Remember also that your body perspective may have changed during your program. Think about how you viewed your body then compared with now. Root your praise and criticism in reality. Above all else, if you've been totally committed to your program, don't forget to praise yourself for your work and dedication.

APPRENTICE WEEK 9

Weights: Day #1...#5

Flat Bench Presses	2	×	12–15
Incline Bench Presses	2	×	12–15
Low-Pulley Row	2	×	15–20
Rear Pull-downs	2	×	15–20
Dumbbell Presses	2	×	12–15
Dumbbell Side Raises	2	×	12–15
Bent-over Side Raises	2	×	12–15
Incline Dumbbell Curls	3	×	12–15
Barbell Curls	3	×	12–15
Push-downs	4	×	15–20
Leg Extensions	2	×	15–20
Leg Presses	2	×	12–15
Lying Leg Curls	3	×	12–15
Hyperextensions	2	×	15–20
Leg-Press Raises	3	×	15–20
Seated Calf Raises	3	×	12–15
Lying Leg Raises	2	×	15–20
Scissors	2	×	12–15
Dumbbell Wrist Curls	4	×	12–15

Weights: Day #3

Incline Bench Presses	2	×	15–20
Incline Dumbbell Flyes	2	×	12–15
Flat Dumbbell Flyes	2	×	12–15
Front Pull-downs	2	×	15–20
Rear Pull-downs	2	×	12–15
Low Pulley Rows	2	×	12–15
Barbell Presses Behind Neck	2	×	15–20
Bent-over Side Raises	2	×	15–20
Barbell Curls	4	×	15–20
Push-downs	3	×	12–15
Lying French Presses	3	×	12–15
Leg Presses	2	×	15–20

Leg Extensions	2	×	12–15
Lying Leg Curls	3	×	15–20
Hyperextensions	2	×	12–15
Standing Calf Raises	4	×	12–15
Crunches	2	×	15–20
Lying Leg Raises	2	×	15–20
Dumbbell Wrist Curls	3	×	15–20

Aerobics: Day #2...#4...#6...#7

Move all four of your aerobics workouts up to thirty minutes and keep your pulse in the range of 70 to 75 percent.

WEEK 10

The last week! Did you ever think it would get here? At this point you should be very pleased with how you're looking and feeling. If you're less than fully pleased with how your flawless body came out, it could relate to one of these two things:

1. **Is it possible that you did not commit 100 percent energy and effort to all of the elements of your program?**
2. **Is it possible that you didn't root your goals sufficiently in reality?**

I'm very confident that you have created dramatic and positive changes in yourself. Now it's time to admit that my goal in having you read this book and go through your program is kind of a selfish one. The selfishness relates to my satisfaction. You see, I get great satisfaction when someone learns about training and fitness. That you've stuck with it and spent nine weeks learning how your body works really gives me pleasure.

How are you going to keep on learning and improving? By being flexible in your approach. What we've covered in this program are the fundamentals. They might be compared to a map and compass that can guide your way;

it's up to you to determine where to go with them. From this point on you must use this knowledge in conjunction with your experience and add variety to your routines. The variety will come from the different exercises, angles and repetitions you use. How variety plays its role in training beyond the apprentice stage gets a thorough discussion in the journeyman-master section.

Even though you're almost at the end of your ten weeks, it should be obvious that I feel it would be to your advantage to continue setting and achieving ten-week fitness program goals.

I want you to really give 100 percent to the next week. But after this week is over, you'll have a decision to make: Where do you go from here? If you decide to begin another ten-week program, do this:

1. **Decide what your new goal is for the ten weeks.**
2. **Go back to the self-analysis preceding Week 5 of the Apprentice Program. Analyze your progress and decide if you need more time in the Apprentice Program. If you do, begin your training at Week 5 and when you get to Week 10 proceed to Week 1 of the Journeyman Program.**

If you decide you're ready to move up now, start at Week 1 of the Journeyman Program. It's up to you to be flexible enough to adjust your strategy to what your needs are.

What happens if you decide that you just want to maintain the progress you've made during your program, but don't want to commit to a new one? You'll need to determine exactly what you want to get out of your workouts and then develop a flexible strategy. Remember that you will get back from your workouts and nutrition only what you put in. If after this week is over you stop working with weights, stop aerobics and go back to the old eating habits, you'll see your gains disappear.

It's possible, however, to maintain a good degree of what you've accomplished with a relatively minimal amount of investment. The minimum amount of time that you can spend in the gym and still maintain some of your gains is two times per week for weight training and three times per week for aerobics.

Your weight workout should at least resemble one of the workouts you did during the first four weeks. It should still be done with focused intensity and perfect form. Keep your exercises balanced so that you're still working all of your body parts. Aerobics should be done for twenty minutes minimum at around a 70 to 75 percent maximum heart rate.

Your nutrition is going to need to remain fairly constant, but you can begin to allow yourself one day each week where you eat whatever you want. Don't make it a binge or starvation day (depending on whether you've been trying to lose or gain weight). Just eat "normal" foods that you might crave, in amounts that make you comfortable. Then the next day get right back on track.

You should still include some visualization and affirmation exercises. These can be useful with any goal you set for yourself. Always project your affirmations in the positive and create them with the assumption that you've already accomplished them.

So there we are. Enjoy your next week. Work out hard and smart. Do your visualizations and affirmations. Follow your eating plan.

The program's not over yet. Keep pushing forward.

TRAINING

Throughout the Apprentice Program, you've been using high-repetition sets on all your exercises. The high reps have a purpose: They build a neurological mind-to-muscle link. Every time you do a repetition you strengthen this link.

I feel strongly that apprentice trainers should always use high reps for at least the first ten weeks of training so the muscles have a higher stimulation rate. The emphasis on high reps also takes the athlete away from the "How much can you bench?" rut that many people get into. A variety of repetitions plays an important part in my training philosophy, but only after the body is "broken in" by high repetitions. If you had begun at Week 1 trying to do sets of four or five reps, you probably would have injured yourself, and you certainly wouldn't have learned to feel the muscles effectively.

High reps are the starting point. Low-rep and medium-rep ranges are added at more advanced levels to give a wider variety of stimulations to a body that has experience developing a mind-to-muscle link.

NUTRITION AND MOTIVATION

All of a sudden you're hit with a massive craving for some junk food. But you know on an intellectual level that if you eat this junk food, more will probably follow and you'll be undermining everything you've accomplished.

How can you get rid of the craving? First, you must understand where the craving is coming from. Is it physiological—in other words, has it been too many hours since your last meal? If it has, then your blood sugar level has probably plummeted and your body is signaling your brain for fuel that will satisfy its need. At this point, food fantasy takes place. You will crave what you have turned to in the past for comfort and satisfaction. If this is the case, you must eat a clean meal right away. Chances are your craving will be gone by the time the meal is finished.

If the craving is psychological, then you must deal with it in different terms. Let's say your belly is full, but you still want that junk food. Whatever its psychological roots are, your mind is rebelling against your goal, and must be stopped. When this happens, stop it with your visualization techniques. Find a quiet place, breathe yourself down and go through the exercise you've been doing. This time, once you step past the doorway of your dreams, see yourself sit down at a table where one of your clean meals sits in front of you. This may sound silly, but watch yourself not only eat it, but enjoy it and feel full and satisfied with it. Now, after the meal, stand up (in your vision) and take off whatever you're wearing. Look at your flawless body from all angles. Tell yourself that eating right makes you look this way and that you like looking this way.

End your visualization in the usual manner. If you do this right and fill it with conviction, emotion, brightness and clarity, your junk-food craving will be gone. You'll be proud that you sat down and solved it instead of running out to satisfy an undermining, temporary whim.

APPRENTICE WEEK 10

Weights: Day #1...#5

Incline Bench Presses	2	×	15–20
Incline Dumbbell Flyes	2	×	12–15
Flat Dumbbell Flyes	2	×	12–15
Front Pull-downs	2	×	15–20
Rear Pull-downs	2	×	12–15

Low-Pulley Rows	2	×	12–15
Barbell Presses Behind Neck	2	×	15–20
Bent-over Side Raises	2	×	15–20
Barbell Curls	4	×	15–20
Push-downs	3	×	12–15
Lying French Presses	3	×	12–15
Leg Presses	2	×	15–20
Leg Extensions	2	×	12–15
Lying Leg Curls	3	×	15–20
Hyperextensions	2	×	12–15
Standing Calf Raises	4	×	12–15
Crunches	2	×	15–20
Lying Leg Raises	2	×	15–20
Dumbbell Wrist Curls	3	×	15–20

Weights: Day #3

Flat Bench Presses	2	×	12–15
Incline Bench Presses	2	×	12–15
Low-Pulley Row	2	×	15–20
Rear Pull-downs	2	×	15–20
Dumbbell Presses	2	×	12–15
Dumbbell Side Raises	2	×	12–15
Bent-over Side Raises	2	×	12–15
Incline Dumbbell Curls	3	×	12–15
Barbell Curls	3	×	12–15
Push-downs	4	×	15–20
Leg Extensions	2	×	15–20
Back Squats	2	×	15–20
Leg Presses	2	×	12–15
Lying Leg Curls	3	×	12–15
Hyperextensions	2	×	15–20
Leg-Press Raises	3	×	15–20
Seated Calf Raises	3	×	12–15
Lying Leg Raises	2	×	15–20
Scissors	2	×	12–15
Barbell Wrist Curls	4	×	12–15

Aerobics: Day #2 . . . #4 . . . #6 . . . #7

Continue the thirty minute workouts, keeping the pulse rate at 75%. Remember to alternate your aerobic workouts to prevent boredom.

The Journeyman
Master Program:
Introduction

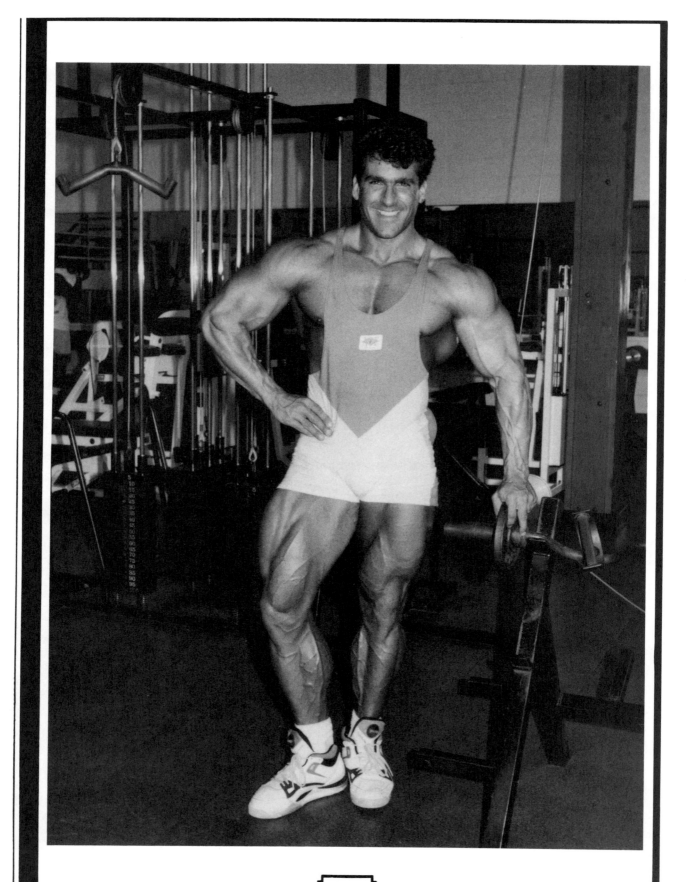

Welcome to the advanced section of *Flawless*. To avoid duplication, I've combined each week's journeyman and master workouts in a single chapter. Since you'll be doing both weights and aerobics on most days, I've combined all the exercises onto one chart. I've also omitted the motivation tips, since the motivation advice presented in the Apprentice Program applies equally to all three programs. (I would, by the way, strongly recommend reading the Apprentice section no matter what level you're at. It's filled with basic information that can be helpful even to experienced trainers.)

The major difference between the journeyman and master levels lies in the workouts themselves. The approach toward training is quite similar; the workouts are simply structured in a way that best advances the goals of each level. The master trainer will be committing more time and days per week to the gym than the journeyman. At the end of each chapter there'll be two different workout sections, one for the journeyman and one for the master.

In order to make this program a success, the first thing I'd like you to do is read through this entire section so that you'll know the direction you're headed in. Then come back to the first week and begin your program. Be sure to fully integrate every element of it. Don't neglect your nutrition or motivational exercises. They're as essential as the actual workouts in attaining your goal of flawlessness.

WEEK 1

At the beginning of this first week, I want you to decide exactly what you want to get out of the program. As an advanced-level trainer, your goal will be rooted in experience. Based on this experience I want you to make a journal entry describing in realistic yet far-reaching terms your goal for the next ten weeks. This is different from the contract you wrote with yourself in the Introduction. This goal description plants an idea deep in your mind—and in your journal—that you can use to guide and reassure yourself throughout the ten weeks.

Don't be afraid to update your overall goal occasionally as the weeks go by. Every week you will have a more experienced perspective, combined with a greater feel for this program. Insights and direction can be fine-tuned in your goal statement. I also hope to persuade those of you who don't like to write to believe in the power of recording your dreams and goals.

During the next seventy days you'll be working with a lot of different training concepts. Some may be new to you. Remember to make this ten-week journey an adventure. You're setting out to do something great—for yourself. Dream big and work hard.

TRAINING #1

There are three key elements that dominate my overall philosophy toward dynamic physical change. These three key elements are balance, variety and feel. Each one integrates with the other two to create an aggressive push toward rapid gains and sustained physical and mental progress. I discussed these elements at length in my previous book, *Beyond Built*, but I'd like to talk more about them, since they underpin every point I'll be making in this section.

By *balance* I mean first the idea of symmetry and proportion. True balance on a bodybuilding level is having all parts developed in proportioned relationship to each other. No single body part should dominate.

I definitely don't subscribe to the school that dictates building only on strengths. Strengths, of course, must be worked, but true physical balance lies in perfecting weaknesses. Experience, a keen eye and intuition will lead you toward your goal if you are open to seeing physical weaknesses not as something to be hidden but rather, as something to be embraced and given priority. A lagging body part presents a challenge. It is a wall that must be gone through, over or around; it must be confronted intelligently and systematically.

I see *variety* as an essential element in every well-planned training strategy. If you do the exact same workout for weeks, months or years on end, you'll become bored, and so will your body. You must train your body with a wide variety of different exercises, angles and repetitions for it to develop to its fullest potential. There is no way around this. In this program you're going to do lots of different exercises and repetition ranges for the muscles.

Of the three key factors, I would have to rank *feel* as the most important. The feel of the muscle during the execution of an exercise is the very foundation of my personal training philosophy. I've already spoken at length about this essential element in "How the Muscles Work." I'd suggest to you that no matter how much experience you have in the gym, you use that section as a reference for perfecting your exercises and their execution.

The bottom line is this: If you don't feel the muscle, any gains you make will be accidental. I don't know about you, but I don't like accidents, and I certainly don't want muscular gains to be a minor side effect of my workouts. I want you to make your training purposeful. In other words, every action and movement you do in the gym should have a purpose, and that purpose should be to accomplish your flawlessness goals. Don't grope around in the dark; make every set and rep you do count. Promise yourself that from this workout on, your focus will be on *feeling* the muscle work, from full extension to full contraction. Make the exercise mean something more than just moving a weight around. Each repetition you do right brings you one step closer to your goal.

Focus in and feel the muscle.

TRAINING #2

Some of you may be wondering, as you read through this book for the first time, why the workouts change so much all the time. Why don't I just do one routine for each body part and use that routine throughout the ten weeks? The reason is that your muscles thrive on change and crawl into a rut when routines remain static for weeks, months or years on end. For my own workouts, I try to change several elements from one training session to the next. Ideally no two body-part workouts will ever be identical. Something should always be changing—the exercises, the rep ranges, the angles, the hand spacing and so on.

Someone who endlessly follows the same routine with the same exercises, angles, reps, etc., is just being lazy. I've watched people get to the point where they could go through their workouts in their sleep. Your muscles and your mind thrive on change. In weight training the common definition of "progressive resistance" is "the body making adaptations to increasingly greater work-loads." There is, however, a second meaning that is often neglected: "*progressively* changing and fighting against the *resistance* to change."

This is why I developed for myself an "armory of exercises" for each body part. Each armory is literally a list of ten to fifteen different exercises for each body part that are rotated in and out of the various routines. The exercises are not unusual; they're the normal ones done with barbells, dumbbells and pulley machines. It is the fact that I utilize a full spectrum of exercises that makes the system so effective.

When you use an "armory" approach it's essential to keep a daily training journal in order to give some sense of order to the whole thing. By the way, here is something I've learned over the years: If there's an exercise in your armory that you keep avoiding (assuming that it does not have an adverse side effect on an injured area), it's probably exactly the one you need.

NUTRITION

As I've said now several times, eating clean foods is essential to your progress. There's one element of nutrition, however, that is often overlooked or neglected. That element is fluid intake. The simple task of drinking water can literally derail your fitness goals, if you don't drink enough, or accelerate your progress toward them. Am I exaggerating? Hardly.

To understand the importance of drinking lots of fluids, you need only examine the percentage of your body that is composed of water. The statistics I've read vary, but generally 70 to 75 percent is in the ballpark. That's a lot of water.

What happens if you don't drink enough fluids? Quite simply, you get dehydrated. When your body is dehydrated your muscles do not function at their peak efficiency, which translates to a decrease in strength, endurance and recuperation.

Also, when the body becomes dehydrated, the mineral (or electrolyte) balance is diminished severely, interfering with nerve impulses, causing severe muscle cramps and leading to possible muscle injuries.

On an athletic diet, the higher protein levels can cause toxins to build up in the kidneys. Large amounts of fluids must be ingested to flush out those toxins and ensure normal function.

What types of fluids are the best and what is the right amount to drink? Far and away the best fluid for athletes is plain water. I also drink iced tea, but in moderation since it's a source of caffeine. I'll drink coffee only early in the day (some time prior to my workout)—also to limit my caffeine intake. I like the new NutraSweet drink mixes, such as Crystal Light and Kool-Aid, because they taste good, contain no sugar and get me to drink my fluid quota.

You see, I have a really bad habit of not drinking enough if I don't pay strict attention. I put a chalkboard in the kitchen and record my daily liquid intake to know if I'm on or off target. For me, it works.

The ideal amount of fluids an athletic person needs is somewhere between one-half and one gallon per day (that's eight to sixteen eight-ounce glasses). When you first begin drinking this much water each day, your bladder will be working overtime. Within a few days, though, it should simmer down. I'd suggest limiting the amount of diet colas consumed in a day, because they're very high in phosphorus. A high phosphorus level will deplete your body's calcium stores, which could lead to severe muscle cramps.

WEEK 1
JOURNEYMAN WORKOUTS

The journeyman workout system will follow the same structure from week to week throughout this program. You will do weight training four days each week and moderate aerobics, as described in "Stretching and Aerobics," five days each week.

The changes that will occur will be in the exercises, angles and repetitions. I describe each week based on Day 1 through Day 7. Day 1 can fall on any day of the week and will depend on what day you begin the program. Once you've established what Day 1 is, stick to that structure throughout the whole ten weeks.

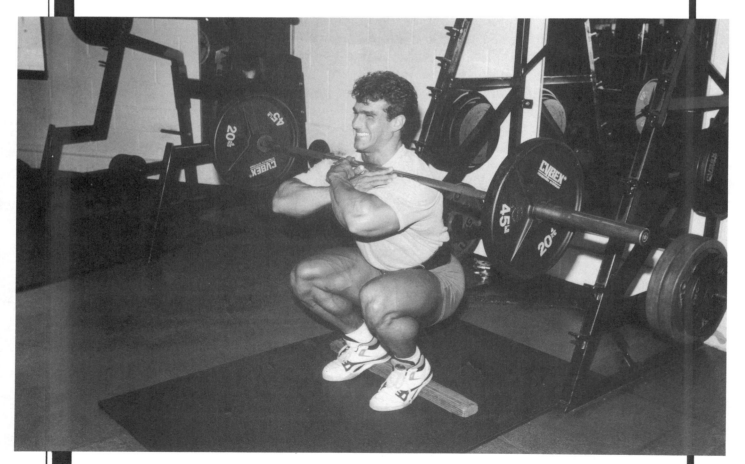

Front Squats are an excellent advanced exercise affecting primarily the quadriceps. The trick is in keeping the bar properly balanced.

The training structure for each week is:

DAY 1
Chest, shoulders, triceps, front thighs, abdominals
Aerobics

DAY 2
Back, biceps, forearms, hamstrings, calves
Aerobics

DAY 3
Rest from weights
Aerobics

DAY 4
Same body parts as Day 1
Aerobics

DAY 5
Same body parts as Day 2
Aerobics

DAY 6
Rest from weights and aerobics

DAY 7
Rest from weights and aerobics

JOURNEYMAN WEEK 1

DAY #1

Incline Bench Press	3	×	6–8
Dips for Chest	3	×	10–12
Flat Dumbbell Flyes	3	×	12–15
Barbell Presses Behind Neck	3	×	12–15
Dumbbell Side Raises	3	×	6–8
Bent-over Pulley Side Raises	3	×	12–15

Push-downs	4	×	10–12
Bench Dips	4	×	12–20
Leg Extensions	4	×	15–20
45-Degree Leg Presses	4	×	12–15
Crunches	3	×	12–15
Lying Leg Raises	3	×	12–15

Aerobics: 20-30 minutes; 70-75% range

Note: Turn to the index to find photos and performance instructions for unfamiliar exercises.

DAY #2

Front Pull-downs	4	×	8–10
Low-Pulley Rows	4	×	6–8
Half Deadlift/Shrugs	3	×	10–12
Barbell Curls	4	×	10–12
Concentration Curls	3	×	12–15
Barbell Wrist Curls	3	×	15–20
Lying Leg Curls	4–5	×	12–20
Standing Calf Raises	3	×	20–25
Seated Calf Raises	3	×	10–12

Aerobics: 20-30 minutes; 70-75% range

DAY #3

Aerobics: 30-40 minutes; 65-70% range

DAY #4

Flat Dumbbell Bench Presses	3	×	8–10
Incline Dumbbell Presses	3	×	6–8
Cable Crossovers	2	×	15–20
Across-Bench Pull-overs	2	×	15–20
Seated Dumbbell Presses	3	×	8–10
Upright Rows	3	×	15–20
Seated Bent-over Side Raises	3	×	6–8
Lying French Presses	4	×	8–10
Overhead Pulley Extensions	4	×	6–8
Back Squats	4	×	8–12
Hack Squats	3	×	12–15
Hanging Leg Raises	3	×	15–25
Frog Kicks	3	×	15–25

Aerobics: 20-30 minutes; 70-75% range

DAY #5

Close-Grip Pull-downs	4	×	12–15
One-Dumbbell Rows	4	×	6–8
Dumbbell Shrugs	3	×	15–20
Hyperextensions	3	×	20–25
Alternating Dumbbell Curls	4	×	6–8
One-Arm Preacher Curls	3	×	8–12
Reverse Curls	3	×	8–10
Standing Leg Curls	4–5	×	15–20
Leg-Press Calf Raise	5–6	×	15–20

Aerobics: 20-30 minutes; 70-75% range

DAY #6..#7
No weights or aerobics.

WEEK 1
MASTER WORKOUTS

Master workouts will follow a day-on, one-day-off pattern throughout the entire program. Therefore, body-part workouts will not necessarily fall on the same day each week, since a complete cycle takes four days to complete.

The body-part breakdown for your training is:

DAY 1
Chest, shoulders, triceps, abdominals
Aerobics

DAY 2
Front thighs, hamstrings, calves
Aerobics

DAY 3
Back, traps/lower back, biceps, forearms
Aerobics

DAY 4
Rest from weights.
Aerobics—Your option; you can rest or do 20–30 minutes.

DAY 5
Repeat Day 1.

DAY 6
Repeat Day 2.

DAY 7
Repeat Day 3.

MASTER WEEK 1

DAY #1

Incline Bench Presses	4	×	6–8
Incline Flyes	4	×	12–15
Flat Dumbbell Presses	3	×	6–8
Across-Bench Pull-overs	3	×	15–20
Dumbbell Side Raises	4	×	10–12
Rear Pulley Crunches	4	×	12–15
Barbell Presses Behind the Neck	4	×	6–8
Bench Dips	4	×	15–20
Push-downs	4	×	6–8
Two-Dumbbell Kickbacks	3	×	10–12
Hanging Leg Raises	3	×	15–20 (tri-set)
Lying Leg Raises	3	×	15–20 (tri-set)
Crunches	3	×	15–20 (tri-set)

Aerobics: 20-30 minutes; 70-75% range

DAY #2

Extensions	4	×	15–20
Front Squats	4	×	12–15
Lunges	4	×	10–12 (each leg)
Lying Leg Curls	4–5	×	12–15 (bi-set)
Stiff-Leg Deadlifts	4–5	×	12–15 (bi-set)
Standing Calf Raises	3–4	×	20–25 (tri-set)
Seated Calf Raises	3–4	×	12–15 (tri-set)
Tibia Raises	3–4	×	20–25 (tri-set)

Aerobics: 30 minutes; 70-75% range

DAY #3

Wide-Grip Pull-downs	4	×	12–15
Close-Grip Pull-downs	4	×	8–10
One-Dumbbell Rows	4	×	10–12
Half Deadlift/Shrugs	3	×	8–10
Hyperextensions	3	×	20–25
Incline Dumbbell Curls	4	×	10–12
Barbell Curls	3–4	×	8–10
One-Arm Pulley Curls	3	×	12–15
Pulley Compound Wrist Curls	3	×	12–15

Aerobics: 30 minutes; 70-75% range

DAY #4

Aerobics: 20-30 minutes; 65-70% range (This is optional. If your body is tired, take a rest from aerobics today.)

DAY #5

Bench Presses	4	×	6–8
Incline Dumbbell Presses	4	×	8–10
Cable Crossovers	3	×	15–20
Across-Bench Pull-overs	3	×	12–15
Dumbbell Presses	4	×	6–8
Seated Bent-over Side Raises	4	×	10–12
Lying Compound Side Raises	4	×	10–12
Rope Push-downs	4	×	6–8
Overhead Pulley Extensions	4	×	12–15
Lying French Presses	3	×	15–20
▌Hanging Leg Raises	3	×	12–15 (tri-set)
▌Lying Leg Raises	3	×	12–15 (tri-set)
▌Twisting Crunches	3	×	12–15 (tri-set)

Aerobics: 30 minutes; 70-75% range

DAY #6

Hack Squats	4	×	12–15
45-Degree Leg Presses	3	×	15–20
Leg Extensions	4	×	15–20
Standing Leg Curls	4	×	12–15
Lying Leg Curls	4	×	10–12
Leg-Press Calf Raises	4	×	20–25
▌Seated Calf Raises	3	×	10–12 (bi-set)
▌Tibia Raises	3	×	15–20 (bi-set)

Aerobics: 30 minutes; 70-75% range

DAY #7

Wide Rear Pull-downs	5	×	15–20
Low-Pulley Rows	4	×	6–8
T-Bar Rows	4	×	8–10
▌Dumbbell Shrugs	4	×	12–15 (bi-set)
▌Hyperextensions	4	×	20–25 (bi-set)
Concentration Curls	4–5	×	10–15
Barbell Preacher Curls	4	×	6–8
Zottman Curls	4	×	12–15
Barbell Wrist Curls	4	×	15–20

Aerobics: 30 minutes; 70-75% range

WEEK 2

As you go into the second week of your program, I want to reinforce the importance of reviewing each week's level of progress, in order to determine whether or not you're on the right track. This concept also reinforces the notion of keeping an accurate training and nutritional journal. For most of you, this training and eating lifestyle represents a priority that may rank below work or personal relationships. Consequently, you may feel I'm putting too much emphasis on journal keeping. I couldn't disagree more. Progress comes when you know where you have been and what you did to get there. The more pertinent details you have, the greater your knowledge and foresight will be.

Remember, too, that this is a learning process. You're learning how your body works, not just with the aim of meeting your ten-week goal, but also with the goal of maintaining permanent flawlessness.

So get into the gym and make the exercises work for you, eat right, visualize and at the end write it all down. Somewhere down the road—it may be next week or next year—you'll be glad you did.

TRAINING #1

Where are you headed with your training? I know that at the moment you're working toward a ten-week goal, and I don't want to steer your attention away from that. I do, however, want to talk about what lies beyond these ten weeks. I don't see this as a distraction from your goal so much as a distinction that could help create a new perspective in how you look at your workouts. You should always be moving toward a greater understanding of where training fits into your life. The more you know about something, such as working out, the more efficiently you can perform that task. Since you're reading this book to expand your training knowledge, you must agree with me.

The point is, I don't want you to remain a slave to a structured fitness plan for the rest of your life. Just as in a science experiment some elements must remain constant in order to determine how variables affect the outcome, so, too, your training needs constant structured workouts in order for you to know how your unique, individual body reacts. But once you know what that reaction is, you can determine if some change might bring you closer to your goal.

My own bodybuilding and fitness goals are constantly changing. There have been times when I've gone along for several years with hard-core competitive bodybuilding as my priority, then a new priority presented itself and I pulled back from that level of commitment, changing my approach to training as well. I followed my instincts to make the adjustment.

You should look at the next ten weeks as a highly structured, goal-oriented period, but you should also look toward a time somewhere down the road when you can break free of the structure. Use your instinct to know exactly what you need, when you need it and how to apply it.

That's how I approach my own training. For years I used structured routines and watched how they affected my body. Because I was tuned into learning what effect my actions were having, I'm now able to intuitively know what my body needs when I walk into the gym. So follow your program to the letter and keep your eyes open to learn what effect the program is having. Use your training journal to record your observations. Trust me: Years from now, when you're trying to recall how you created the success that you did, you'll be glad that you wrote it all down.

TRAINING #2

There are dozens of ways to combine body parts when doing a split-routine. Over the years I've tried them all and, at the moment, I find the split-system used in these routines to be the most efficient. The reason is recovery. Muscle recovery after a workout dictates our training structures nearly as much as the exercises themselves. The workout structure should try to take this into account. This system also takes into account the primary and secondary muscle groups that work in conjunction with each other. (I discussed primary and secondary muscles at length in "How the Muscles Work.")

For example, the triceps and deltoid function as secondary muscles when a chest-pressing movement is done. Even though you should be trying to isolate the chest as much as possible on a press, it's not structurally possible. The triceps and deltoids will always get some work. Since the triceps and deltoids are already warmed up by this secondary work on compound chest movements, why not train them in the same workout?

Do you see why this would make the workout more efficient? Basically, since triceps and deltoids will already be slightly worked, fewer isolating primary sets will be necessary to take those two body parts to the "diminishing pump" level. Also, since the chest, triceps and deltoid system is worked in one day, it's allowed complete rest until the next workout. Far greater recovery takes place and, in turn, faster gains are realized. This applies equally to the back, biceps, and rear-deltoid/trap system.

In the journeyman workout, the hamstrings are linked with the back because of their secondary and symbiotic relationship to lower-back work. It also seems logical to me to work the "upper" (arm) and "lower" (leg) biceps on the same day, given their structural similarities.

What you'll achieve by following this scheme is a fully integrated, intense workout that afterward leaves the affected body parts "untouched" for an ideal recuperation period.

NUTRITION

What about supplements? We all know the range of bodybuilding and health supplements that fill the shelves of vitamin stores and the advertising pages of bodybuilding magazines.

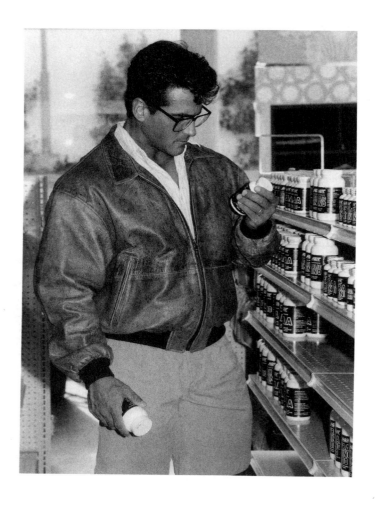

How many of these products are worth your money and how many are worthless junk? Well, I can answer the "worthless junk" part in this way: Companies that manufacture supplements for bodybuilders are trying to make money. For most companies the bottom line is profit—the margin between how cheaply a product can be made and the price that can be charged to the consumer. Usually the margin is quite large. A great deal of money is also invested in advertising the tremendous benefits that can be derived from the use of such products. Wild exaggerations have definitely been made about products that may only *marginally* help the user to achieve greater development. *Caution:* The wilder an advertisement's claim, the greater chance that the product is fraudulent.

I can think of one company (I won't name it) that takes out glossy multi-page ads in all the biggest bodybuilding magazines, making wild claims about the benefits derived from the use of its *very expensive* system of supplementation. The ads come complete with testimonials—even a pro bodybuilder's claim that it was these products alone that created the body he now has.

Now I do bodybuilding seminars all over the world and have spoken to literally hundreds of this name brand's users. Out of those hundreds, only five have expressed satisfaction with the changes associated with use of this complex assortment of esoteric supplements. Most spoke of feeling ripped off. The moral is: When it comes to nutrition supplements, "Let the buyer beware."

There are some companies, of course, that have a high level of integrity and manufacture a good line of basic supplements that don't make extraordinary claims. In next week's nutrition section I'll talk about which supplements *should* fit into your program.

JOURNEYMAN WEEK 2

DAY #1

Incline Bench Presses	3	×	6–8
Dips for Chest	3	×	10–12
Flat Flyes	3	×	12–15
Barbell Presses Behind the Neck	3	×	12–15
Dumbbell Side Raises	3	×	6–8
Bent-over Pulley Side Raises	3	×	12–15
Push-downs	4	×	10–12
Bench Dips	4	×	12–20
Leg Extensions	4	×	15–20
45-Degree Leg Presses	4	×	12–15
Crunches	3	×	15–25
Lying Leg Raises	3	×	15–25

Aerobics: 20-30 minutes; 70-75% range

DAY #2

Wide Front Pull-downs	4	×	8–10
Low-Pulley Rows	4	×	6–8
Half Deadlift/Shrugs	3	×	10–12
Barbell Curls	4	×	10–12
Concentration Curls	3	×	12–15
Barbell Wrist Curls	3	×	15–20
Lying Leg Curls	4–5	×	12–20
Standing Calf Raises	3	×	20–25
Seated Calf Raises	3	×	10–12

Aerobics: 20-30 minutes; 70-75% range

DAY #3

Aerobics: 30-40 minutes; 65-70% range

DAY #4

Flat Dumbbell Bench Presses	3	×	8–10
Incline Dumbbell Presses	3	×	6–8
Cable Crossovers	2	×	15–20
Across-Bench Pullovers	2	×	15–20
Seated Dumbbell Presses	3	×	8–10
Upright Rows	3	×	15–20
Seated Bent-over Side Raises	3	×	6–8
Lying French Presses	4	×	8–10
Overhead Pulley Extensions	4	×	6–8
Back Squats	4	×	8–12
Hack Squats	3	×	12–15
Hanging Leg Raises	3	×	15–25
Frog Kicks	3	×	15–25

Aerobics: 20-30 minutes; 70-75% range

DAY #5

Close-Grip Pulldowns	4	×	12–15
One-Dumbbell Rows	4	×	6–8
Dumbbell Shrugs	3	×	15–20
Hyperextensions	3	×	20–25
Alternating Dumbbell Curls	4	×	6–8
One-Arm Preacher Curls	3	×	8–12
Reverse Curls	3	×	8–10
Standing Leg Curls	4–5	×	15–20
Leg-Press Calf Raises	5–6	×	15–20

Aerobics: 20-30 minutes; 70-75% range

DAY #6 . . . #7

No weights or aerobics.

MASTER WEEK 2

DAY #1

Aerobics: 20-30 minutes; 65-70% range (If your body is tired, take a rest from aerobics today.)

DAY #2

Incline Bench Presses	4	×	6–8
Incline Flyes	4	×	12–15
Flat Dumbbell Presses	3	×	6–8
Across-Bench Pull-overs	3	×	15–20
Dumbbell Side Raises	4	×	10–12
Rear Pulley Crunches	4	×	12–15
Barbell Presses Behind the Neck	4	×	6–8
Bench Dips	4	×	15–20
Push-downs	4	×	6–8
Two Dumbbell Kickbacks	3	×	10–12
▎Hanging Leg Raises	3	×	15–20 (tri-set)
▎Lying Leg Raises	3	×	15–20 (tri-set)
▎Crunches	3	×	15–20 (tri-set)

Aerobics: 30 minutes; 70-75% range

DAY #3

Extensions	4	×	15–20
Front Squats	4	×	12–15
Lunges	4	×	10–12
▎Lying Leg Curls	4–5	×	12–15 (bi-set)
▎Stiff-Leg Deadlifts	4–5	×	12–15 (bi-set)
▎Standing Calf Raises	3–4	×	20–25 (tri-set)
▎Seated Calf Raises	3–4	×	12–15 (tri-set)
▎Tibia Raises	3–4	×	20–25 (tri-set)

Aerobics: 30 minutes; 70-75% range

DAY #4

Wide-Grip Pull-downs	4	×	12–15
Close-Grip Pull-downs	4	×	8–10
One-Dumbbell Rows	4	×	10–12
Half-Deadlift/Shrugs	3	×	8–10
Hyperextensions	3	×	20–25
Incline Dumbbell Curls	4	×	10–12
Barbell Curls	3–4	×	8–10
One-Arm Pulley Curls	3	×	12–15
Pulley Compound Wrist Curls	3	×	12–15

Aerobics: 30 minutes; 70-75% range

DAY #5
Aerobics: 20-30 minutes; 65-70% range (This is optional. If your body is tired, take a rest from aerobics today.)

DAY #6

Bench Presses	4	×	6–8
Incline Dumbbell Presses	4	×	8–10
Cable Crossovers	3	×	15–20
Across-Bench Pull-overs	3	×	12–15
Dumbbell Presses	4	×	6–8
Seated Bent-over Side Raises	4	×	10–12
Lying Compound Side Raises	4	×	10–12
Rope Push-downs	4	×	6–8
Overhead Pulley Extensions	4	×	12–15
Lying French Presses	3	×	15–20
▌Hanging Leg Raises	3	×	15–25 (tri-set)
▌Lying Leg Raises	3	×	15–25 (tri-set)
▌Twisting Crunches	3	×	15–25 (tri-set)

Aerobics: 30 minutes; 70-75% range

DAY #7

Hack Squats	4	×	12–15
45-Degree Leg Presses	3	×	15–20
Extensions	4	×	15–20
Standing Leg Curls	4	×	12–15
Lying Leg Curls	4	×	10–12
Leg-Press Calf Raises	4	×	20–25
▌Seated Calf Raises	3	×	10–12 (bi-set)
▌Tibia Raises	3	×	15–20 (bi-set)

Aerobics: 30 minutes; 70-75% range

WEEK 3

Now that you've successfully completed two weeks of your program, I want you to make a complete analysis of your body's strengths and weaknesses (the same analysis that I had apprentice trainers complete early in their program). This analysis should be very honest, but not an excuse for bashing yourself over perceived flaws. We all have a structure we're born with. Creating a flawless body is not only improving what is changeable, but also accepting what is not.

By now you should have two weeks of solid journal entries. At the start of your third week, start a blank page and draw a line from top to bottom down the middle. On top of the left-hand column write "Strengths" and at the right "Weaknesses." Now, in a place where you can have complete privacy, strip off all your clothes. Stand in front of a full-length mirror and really look. Let your eyes open and take in the full scope of what your body really looks like, from the front, sides and rear; top to bottom. Record what you see.

Next to everything you list as a weakness, write a short goal-oriented sentence on how that aspect of your body can be improved. Keep it positive and rooted in reality.

Use the mirror analysis sessions from time to time throughout your program to monitor your progress and also to learn a higher level of acceptance of the body you were gifted with.

"Knowledge is Power."

TRAINING

I talk a great deal about the importance of exercise perfection in bodybuilding and how perfect form combined with squeezing the muscles creates the greatest opportunity for progress. There is, however, one more factor to consider in the formula for creating the perfect set. That factor is intensity.

What exactly is intensity as it relates to your workouts? Training intensity is an extreme mental and physical focus directed into the set you're performing. High intensity is carrying a set to the point where no more repetitions can be done. This is where a huge gray area arises and the individual is required to make a judgment call to get the whole concept fine-tuned. Because the line between high intensity and overtraining shifts from workout to workout, complete knowledge of your own body becomes essential.

It's not always the hardest-training athlete who gets the best results. The smart athlete, who combines hard work with intelligent and intuitive knowledge, will get the gains every time.

The balancing act comes in knowing the exact amount of sets and exercises that will have to be done for a body part to make it grow and still allow sufficient recuperation before the next workout. What are the physical signals that can give you an idea when a body part has had enough?

Generally speaking, you can monitor the volume of a body-part workout according to the pump you feel in the muscle. In most cases a body-part workout should be concluded just past the point where the maximum pump (fullness and tightness caused by blood filling the muscle) begins to diminish— the "diminishing pump" concept we saw earlier. So you can, by observation, adjust your body-part set and exercise volume according to this indicator.

The point of diminishing pump will probably come in slightly different places from workout to workout, but after a while you'll be able to intuitively know when you're reaching the best point to finish a body part and move on. Once again, your journal can be extraordinarily helpful in providing you with insight, after the fact, on the average number of sets it takes you to get to a level of diminishing pump. Some of the factors that will figure into your ideal workout volume will be:

1. The actual intensity with which you perform the sets during the workout.
2. If you're taking the exercises to positive failure or beyond.
3. How well the muscle has recuperated from the last time it was worked.
4. How disciplined you've been with your nutrition.
5. The amount of mental baggage you bring with you to the gym.
6. The quality and quantity of sleep prior to a workout.

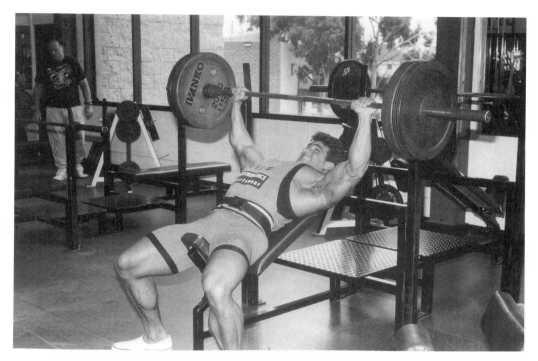

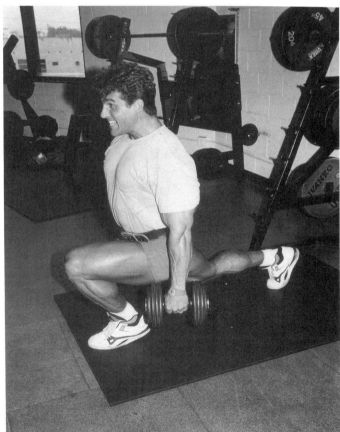

Lunges will help those at the master level cut up their thighs and glutes. They can be performed either with dumbbells, as pictured here, or with a barbell.

NUTRITION

My own opinion of supplements has not changed much in several years. I'm a big believer in the basics. If you're looking for some miracle to happen by taking a natural nutrition supplement, you're probably going to be disappointed. Any supplementation you use should be there only to reinforce your core nutrition program.

My own supplement program revolves around these products:

1. A strong multivitamin and mineral—This should be broken up into incremental doses throughout the day and taken with each meal.

2. Extra multiminerals—I take these prior to and just after any type of training to replace minerals lost through muscle contraction and sweat.

3. Liver Tablets—To me this is the ultimate endurance supplement. The vitamin B properties of liver help the body use its glycogen more efficiently. I take several desiccated, defatted liver tabs with each meal and before and after workouts.

4. Balanced multi-amino acids—I take aminos with all my meals and especially before and after training (I'll devote an entire nutrition tip to this later). A balanced multi-amino should have a spectrum that resembles the amino profile of a gram of egg-white protein.

5. Branch-chain amino acids—The key aminos that need replenishment just after the workout are leucine, isoleucine and valine—the branch-chain aminos. In addition to my regular aminos, I take branch-chain aminos just before the workout and along with the small carb meal immediately after an intense workout. Replacing branch-chains will greatly enhance your body's ability to recuperate from a workout.

6. Quality protein powder—I use protein powder only as a supplement when I'm trying to consume more calories than I could possibly eat in solid food and when I'm eating on the run, as an occasional meal replacement. To bring a protein drink into balance, I'll mix in fruit to add carbohydrates. But I do not rely on powders as a mainstay of my nutrition plan, and you shouldn't either.

In next week's nutrition tips, I'll talk about a few supplements that I add to my regimen prior to competition and that you might benefit from during your program.

JOURNEYMAN WEEK 3

DAY #1

Flat Barbell Bench Presses	3	×	6–8
Incline Flyes	3	×	12–15
▌ Dips for Chest	2–3	×	8–10 (bi-set)
▌ Across-Bench Pullovers	2–3	×	8–10 (bi-set)
One-Arm Pulley Side Raises	3	×	12–15
Incline Side Raises	3	×	8–10
Seated Dumbbell Presses	3	×	15–20
One-Arm Push-downs	4	×	12–15
Two-Dumbbell Kickbacks	4	×	8–10
Leg Extensions	4	×	10–12
Hack Squats	4	×	15–20
Leg Raises	3	×	12–15
Scissors	3	×	12–15
Crunches	3	×	15–25

Aerobics: 20-30 minutes; 70-75% range

DAY #2

Wide Rear Pull-downs	3	×	6–8
Low-Pulley Rows	3	×	15–20
One-Dumbbell Rows	3	×	8–10
▌ Barbell Shrugs	2–3	×	12–15 (bi-set)
▌ Hyperextensions	2–3	×	15–20 (bi-set)
Incline Dumbbell Curls	3	×	10–12
Barbell Preacher Curls	3	×	12–15
Two-Dumbbell Wrist Curls	3	×	12–15
Standing Leg Curls	3	×	8–12
Lying Leg Curls	2	×	15–20
Standing Calf Raises	3	×	15–20
Seated Calf Raises	3	×	15–20

Aerobics: 25-30 minutes; 75% range

DAY #3

Aerobics: 35-40 minutes; 65-70% range

DAY #4

Flat Flyes	3	×	10–12
Incline Dumbbell Presses	3	×	10–12
Incline Flyes	4	×	8–10
Seated Presses Behind the Neck	3	×	6–8
Pulley Upright Rows	3	×	8–10
Seated Bent-over Side Raises	3	×	15–20

Reverse-Grip Push-downs	4	×	6–8
Bench Dips	4	×	12–15
Back Squats	4	×	6–8
Leg Presses	2	×	12–15
Leg Extensions	2	×	15–20
Twisting Crunches	5	×	15–20

Aerobics: 25-30 minutes; 75% range

DAY #5

Pull-ups to Front	4	×	8–12
T-Bar Rows	4	×	10–15
Half Deadlift/Shrugs	3	×	15–20
One-Arm Preacher Curls	4	×	6–8
Barbell Curls	4	×	8–10
Reverse Curls	3	×	12–15
Lying Leg Curls	4–5	×	8–15
Leg-Press Raises	3	×	10–12
Seated Calf Raises	3	×	10–12

Aerobics: 25-30 minutes; 75% range

DAY #6 ... #7

Aerobics: 35-40 minutes; 65-70% range

MASTER WEEK 3

DAY #1

Wide-Grip Pull-downs	4	×	12–15
Close-Grip Pull-downs	4	×	8–10
One-Dumbbell Rows	4	×	10–12
Half Deadlift/Shrugs	3	×	8–10
Hyperextensions	3	×	20–25
Incline Dumbbell Curls	4	×	10–12
Barbell Curls	3–4	×	8–10
One-Arm Pulley Curls	3	×	12–15
Pulley Compound Wrist Curls	3	×	12–15

Aerobics: 30 minutes; 70-75% range

DAY #2

Incline Dumbbell Curls	4	×	10–12
Barbell Curls	3–4	×	8–10
One-Arm Pulley Curls	3	×	12–15
Pulley Compound Wrist Curls	3	×	12–15

Aerobics: 30 minutes; 70–75% range (This is optional. If your body is tired, take a rest from aerobics today.)

DAY #3

Flat Barbell Bench Presses	4	×	6–8
Incline Barbell Bench Presses	4	×	6–8
▌Incline Flyes	3	×	15–20
▌Cable Crossovers	2	×	12–15 (bi-set)
Across-Bench Pull-overs	2	×	10–12 (bi-set)
One-Arm Pulley Side Raises	4	×	12–15
Seated Dumbbell Presses	3	×	6–8
Bent-over Dumbbell Side Raises	3	×	8–10
Lying Compound Side Raises	3	×	10–12
Overhead Pulley Extensions	4	×	12–15
Lying Barbell Kickbacks	4	×	8–10
One-Arm Push-downs	4	×	6–8
Crunches	5	×	15–20
Hanging Leg Raises	4	×	15–20

Aerobics: 30-35 minutes; 75-80% range

DAY #4

Standing Leg Curls	4–5	×	15–20
Lying Leg Curls	4–5	×	12–15
Lunges	4	×	10–12
45-Degree Leg Presses	4	×	15–25
Leg Extensions	5	×	8–15
Leg-Press Calf Raises	4	×	15–20
▌Donkey Calf Raises	4	×	12–15 (bi-set)
▌Tibia Raises	4	×	20–25 (bi-set)

Aerobics: 30-35 minutes; 70-75% range

DAY #5

Wide Front Pull-ups	4	×	10–15
Barbell Rows	3	×	8–10
One-Dumbbell Rows	3	×	6–8
Wide Rear Pull-downs	3	×	15–20
Dumbbell Half Deadlift/Shrugs	4–5	×	10–12

Incline Dumbbell Curls	3	×	10–12 (tri-set)
Barbell Curls	3	×	10–12 (tri-set)
Barbell Preacher Curls	3	×	10–12 (tri-set)
Pulley Compound Wrist Curls	4	×	12–15

Aerobics: 30-35 minutes; 75-80% range

DAY #6

Aerobics: Do your aerobics for 30 to 35 minutes in a 75–80% range. (This is optional. If your body is tired, take a rest from aerobics today.)

DAY #7

Incline Dumbbell Presses	4	×	8–10
Flat Dumbbell Presses	4	×	8–10
Dips for Chest	3	×	10–12
Across-Bench Pull-overs	3	×	15–20
Seated Dumbbell Side Raises	3	×	12–15 (bi-set)
Presses Behind the Neck	3	×	12–15 (bi-set)
Rear Pulley Crunches	4	×	8–10
Alternating Fronts			
Dumbbell Raises	3	×	6–8
Push-downs	3–4	×	10–12 (tri-set)
Bench Dips	3–4	×	10–12 (tri-set)
Lying French Presses	3–4	×	10–12 (tri-set)
Lying Leg Raises	3	×	15–25 (tri-set)
Scissors	3	×	10–12 (tri-set)
Twisting Crunches	3	×	15–25 (tri-set)

Aerobics: 30-35 minutes; 70-75% range

WEEK 4

Here you are at the fourth week of your program. Twenty-one days have now been systematically invested in creating not only the body that you want, but also greater health and self-esteem.

I like to use *my* training as time when I can totally escape and spend two hours being totally self-indulgent. Training and eating right just make me feel better about myself. And I know one thing for certain: When I feel good about myself, the overall quality of my life just soars.

Focus in and keep pushing!

TRAINING

You'll notice that your routines are going to encompass a fairly broad range of repetitions. For the most part the rep range runs from six reps as a minimum up to twenty-five as a maximum. This range contradicts a lot of what you'll read about bodybuilding training. For the most part a range of eight-to-twelve reps is pushed almost like a dogmatic religion. My experience has shown that the body needs a much greater variety of reps than the limited eight-to-twelve range provides.

For full development, you're going to need to do intense, heavy, positive-failure sets in the low (six to nine), medium (ten to fifteen) and high (sixteen to twenty-five) repetition ranges. Each of these ranges has a slightly different effect on the muscle fibers and their connective tissues. You would only be slowing your own progress by avoiding any of these low, medium or high ranges.

Remember, high reps shouldn't necessarily mean "light" weights, unless the weight you use won't allow you to achieve positive failure inside your goal rep range.

High reps hurt. They burn like hell and are extremely productive when done right. Keep the weight and intensity high and push yourself through to *physical* positive failure. Don't just stop when the burn gets to be too much for your mind to handle. Block it out by focusing into the muscle and the reps. Don't mistake high reps for fast reps, either. You should be squeezing every rep just as hard on a set of twenty as on a set of ten.

Sets where the repetitions fall below six don't really contribute to your bodybuilding goals, since extremely low reps rely primarily on connective tissue and only secondarily on muscle fibers.

The rep schemes in the routines you'll be encountering here are designed with full development in mind. I'm giving you the benefit of my own years of trial and error in these routines. For maximum results, stick with the rep ranges I've stipulated.

NUTRITION

In addition to my usual lineup of basic supplements, there are two that I use to boost progress during precontest phases. Since this ten-week program is viewed by many as a "peaking" phase, I wanted to include them:

L-Carnitine: I find this supplement very useful when my calories are low. Basically I find that L-Carnitine, taken with meals and just after a workout, helps me maintain lean body mass during times when I'm trying to burn fat and get cut-up. L-Carnitine has been shown to transport long-chain fatty acids into the section of the cell where they're oxidized and most efficiently burned. In other words, fat is more actively converted to usable energy, and therefore all other calories consumed can be utilized for lean-mass maintenance, even if few calories are being eaten.

Chromium: I find that by using a moderate level of chromium, especially just before my workout, my blood sugar stays extremely stable throughout the day. My energy level also stays high and consistent during training. My blood sugar stability becomes crucial during peaking periods. For me, low blood sugar often means dizzy and spaced-out feelings, followed by intense junk-food cravings. So I'm consistent with my five or six meals each day and use a chromium supplement to keep my blood sugar levels stable.

JOURNEYMAN WEEK 4

DAY #1

Flat Barbell Bench Presses	3	×	6–8
Incline Flyes	3	×	12–15
▌Dips for Chest	2–3	×	8–10 (bi-set)
▌Across-Bench Pull-overs	2–3	×	8–10 (bi-set)
One-Arm Pulley Side Raises	3	×	12–15
Incline Side Raises	3	×	8–10
Seated Dumbbell Presses	3	×	15–20
One-Arm Push-downs	4	×	12–15
Two-Dumbbell Kickbacks	4	×	8–10
Leg Extensions	4	×	10–12
Hack Squats	4	×	15–20
▌Leg Raises	3	×	15–25 (tri-set)
▌Scissors	3	×	15–25 (tri-set)
▌Crunches	3	×	15–25 (tri-set)

Aerobics: 20-30 minutes; 70-75% range

DAY #2

Wide Rear Pull-downs	3	×	6–8
Low-Pulley Rows	3	×	15–20
One-Dumbbell Rows	3	×	8–10
▌Barbell Shrugs	2–3	×	12–15 (bi-set)
▌Hyperextensions	2–3	×	15–20 (bi-set)
Incline Dumbbell Curls	3	×	10–12
Barbell Preacher Curls	3	×	12–15
Two-Dumbbell Wrist Curls	3	×	12–15
Standing Leg Curls	3	×	8–12

Lying Leg Curls	2	×	15–20
Standing Calf Raises	3	×	15–20
Seated Calf Raises	3	×	15–20

Aerobics: 25-30 minutes; 75% range

DAY #3

Aerobics: 35-40 minutes; 65-70% range

DAY #4

Flat Flyes	3	×	10–12 (bi-set)
Incline Dumbbell Presses	3	×	10–12 (bi-set)
Incline Flyes	4	×	8–10
Seated Presses Behind the Neck	3	×	6–8
Pulley Upright Rows	3	×	8–10
Seated Bent-over Side Raises	3	×	15–20
Reverse-Grip Push-downs	4	×	6–8
Bench Dips	4	×	12–15
Back Squats	4	×	6–8
Leg Presses	2	×	12–15
Leg Extensions	2	×	15–20
Twisting Crunches	5	×	15–25

Aerobics: 25-30 minutes; 75% range

DAY #5

Pull-ups to Front	4	×	8–12
T-Bar Rows	4	×	10–15
Half Deadlift/Shrugs	3	×	15–20
One-Arm Preacher Curls	4	×	6–8
Barbell Curls	4	×	8–10
Reverse Curl	3	×	12–15
Lying Leg Curls	4–5	×	8–15
Leg-Press Raises	3	×	10–12
Seated Calf Raises	3	×	10–12

Aerobics: 25-30 minutes; 75% range

DAY #6...#7

No weights or aerobics.

MASTER WEEK 4

DAY #1

Back Squats	4	×	6–8
▌Extensions	3	×	15–20 (tri-set)
▌Hack Squats	3	×	12–15 (tri-set)
▌Sissy Squats	3	×	12–15 (tri-set)
▌Lying Leg Curls	4–5	×	12–15 (bi-set)
▌Stiff-Leg Deadlifts	4–5	×	8–10 (bi-set)
▌Standing Calf Raises	3	×	20–30 (tri-set)
▌Seated Calf Raises	3	×	20–30 (tri-set)
▌Tibia Raises	3	×	20–25 (tri-set)

Aerobics: 30-35 minutes; 75-80% range

DAY #2

Wide Rear Pull-ups	4	×	10–12
Wide Front Pull-downs	3	×	6–8
T-Bar Rows	3	×	8–10
Straight-Arm Pull-ins	3	×	12–15
Barbell Shrugs	4	×	15–20
Hyperextensions	4	×	20–25
Standing Alternating Dumbbell Curls	4	×	10–12
One-Arm Preacher Curls	3	×	12–15
Concentration Curls	3	×	6–8
▌Zottman Curls	3	×	12–15 (bi-set)
▌Two-Dumbbell Wrist Curls	3	×	12–15 (bi-set)

Aerobics: 30-35 minutes; 70-75% range

DAY #3

Aerobics: 35-40 minutes; 65-70% range (This is optional. If your body is tired, take a rest from aerobics today.)

DAY #4

Flat Barbell Bench Presses	4	×	6–8
Incline Barbell Bench Presses	4	×	6–8
Incline Flyes	3	×	15–20
▌Cable Crossovers	2	×	12–15 (bi-set)
▌Across-Bench Pull-overs	2	×	10–12 (bi-set)
One-Arm Pulley Side Raises	3	×	12–15
Seated Dumbbell Presses	3	×	6–8
Bent-over Dumbbell Side Raises	3	×	8–10
Lying Compound Side Raises	3	×	10–12
Overhead Pulley Extensions	4	×	12–15

▮ Lying Barbell Kickbacks	4	×	8–10 (bi-set)
▮ One-arm Push-downs	4	×	6–8 (bi-set)
Crunches	5	×	15–20
Hanging Leg Raises	4	×	15–20

Aerobics: 30-35 minutes; 75-80% range

DAY #5

Standing Leg Curls	4–5	×	15–20
Lying Leg Curls	4–5	×	12–15
Lunges	4	×	10–12
45-Degree Leg Presses	4	×	15–25
Leg Extensions	5	×	8–15
Leg-Press Calf Raises	4	×	15–20
▮ Donkey Calf Raises	4	×	12–15 (bi-set)
▮ Tibia Raises	4	×	20–25 (bi-set)

Aerobics: 30-35 minutes; 70-75% range

DAY #6

Wide Front Pull-ups	4	×	10–15
Barbell Rows	3	×	8–10
One-Dumbbell Rows	3	×	6–8
Wide Rear Pull-downs	3	×	15–20
Dumbbell Half Deadlift/Shrugs	4–5	×	10–12
▮ Incline Dumbbell Curls	3	×	10–12 (tri-set)
▮ Barbell Curls	3	×	10–12 (tri-set)
▮ Barbell Preacher Curls	3	×	10–12 (tri-set)
Pulley Compound Wrist Curls	4	×	12–15

Aerobics: 30-35 minutes; 75-80% range

DAY #7

Aerobics: 35-40 minutes; 65-70% range (This is optional. If your body is tired, take a rest from aerobics today.)

SELF-EVALUATION (PRIOR TO WEEK 5)

Before you begin your fifth week, I want you to evaluate your progress. The point of this evaluation is to determine if you're training at the correct experience level. I want you to take this evaluation seriously and definitely base it in reality. If you are on the Journeyman Program, it won't do any good to move to the Master Program before your body has a chance to adapt to its present workload.

The possible program changes resulting from this evaluation are:

1. You're on the Journeyman Program but would be better served by the Apprentice Program.

2. You're on the Journeyman Program, but would actually make faster progress on the Master Program.

3. You are on the Master Program, but would be better suited to the Journeyman Program.

When making your evaluation, use your journal notes, your observations and your experience to answer the following questions:

1. How well has my body adapted to this level?

2. How well are my muscles recovering after each workout?

3. Am I comfortable enough with my current knowledge to move up a level, or should I stay where I am and gain experience?

4. Since a more advanced program involves a greater time commitment, can I realistically make this investment?

(The next three questions cover the intelligent use of intensity in your workouts. They're intended to determine if you are working out at optimum intensity on your current program.)

5. Are the workouts too hard, too easy or just right?

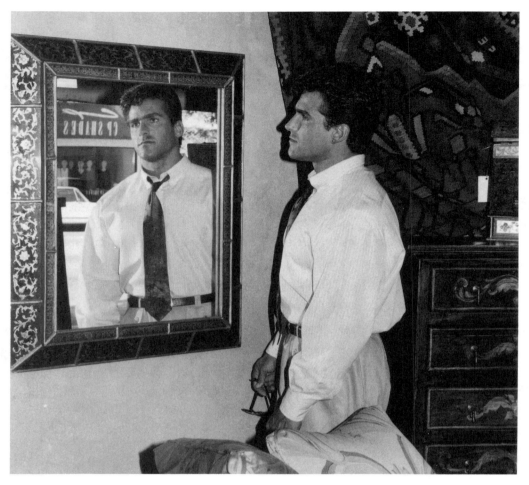

In evaluating yourself, be honest about what you see in the mirror.

6. If they're too easy, am I doing everything possible to work at a high intensity level?

7. If they're too hard, am I abusing the principles that are designed to take an exercise past positive failure, such as forced reps, etc...?

By providing honest and realistic answers to these questions, you'll be able to make an intelligent decision about the next six weeks. Seventy-five percent of the time, I recommend that people stay with the program they've begun. This evaluation is here for the 25 percent whose progress may be advanced by a program-level adjustment.

WEEK 5

At the end of this week, you'll be at the midway point in your program. If you had to rate the consistent effort you've given to this program on a scale of 0 to 100 percent, where would you place yourself? If your effort is 100 percent, you should be seeing and feeling great return on your investment. Remember that this whole training and eating-right business is not something at which you can cheat. You'll be rewarded in direct proportion to the commitment you invest.

Consistent effort is the key. The childhood tale of the hare and the tortoise holds the moral: Steady effort, gaining momentum wherever possible, will over the long run enable you to win the race.

TRAINING

I don't know of any better way to make the muscles visually harder looking or to increase the mind-to-muscle link than flexing a body part between sets. If you're working biceps, for example, don't just stand or sit around in between sets—flex and squeeze your biceps muscles. You'll not only keep your mind focused into the workout by flexing the body part between sets, you'll also open up nerve pathways that will make every repetition you do more effective. Top bodybuilders have known of and employed this practice for years. It is called iso-tension in the magazines, and you can do it for every body part. I know that I would never skip doing it, unless I wanted to hold myself back from making progress.

NUTRITION

What is my view on red meat as a part of the flawlessness nutrition plan? Very favorable—though there's a catch! It can't be just any red meat. If you look at the caloric breakdowns in the nutrition section's overall food list, you'll see a footnote added to round and flank steaks. You'll also see that my beef calorie listing is only five calories per ounce higher than turkey or chicken breast. How is this? Selection and preparation are the answers.

First you must select the right piece of meat (flank and round are the leanest), with as little visible fat showing as possible. Some stores just have fatter beef than others. Believe it or not, to most people higher fat content is desirable: fat adds to the taste. Those people obviously aren't aiming for a flawless body.

Second, don't buy any type of preprepared ground beef, no matter how lean it's supposed to be. I want you to make your own ground beef, and it will be quantum leaps leaner.

When you get a piece of round or flank, do surgery on it. I mean, go at it with a knife and pare away any visible fat. If it's white, cut it away and toss it. Now cut the meat into small cubes. Examine and trim fat from these cubes, then put the cubes into a food processor and grind the meat to a very fine texture. If you want to make patties from this ground beef, make them very thin and grill or broil them so that any remaining fat will drip out.

I like to use a nonstick skillet and cook the meat over medium-high heat, loose (like you're browning meat for sloppy joes or spaghetti sauce) and breaking the clumps up with a spatula until it's done medium-rare. That's my own taste—but you should know that this highly lean beef will dry out the more well-done it gets.

Whether in patty form or loose, I'll then pat and drain the meat with a paper towel to further remove fat. You can add onions and/or sauté with spices. The meat may seem dry, but I usually moisten it with low-sodium salsa or a small amount of low-calorie catsup.

I like beef because my body reacts very favorably to its protein composition. I can only explain it this way—I feel stronger and more energetic when I include lean beef as an animal protein source. I also know that a lot of other very experienced bodybuilders agree with me.

If you don't eat beef for philosophical or other reasons, you certainly won't be holding yourself back by abstaining. I just find that beef gives me an edge.

JOURNEYMAN WEEK 5

DAY #1

Incline Bench Presses	3	×	6–8
Flat Dumbbell Presses	3	×	10–12
Cable Crossovers on Machine	3	×	15–20
▌Seated Dumbbell Side Raises	3	×	10–12 (tri-set)
▌Seated Barbell Presses Behind Neck	3	×	10–12 (tri-set)
▌Seated Bent-over Side Raises	3	×	10–12 (tri-set)
Push-downs	4	×	10–12
Bench Dips	4	×	12–20
Hack Squats	3	×	15–20
45-Degree Leg Presses	3	×	12–15
Leg Extensions	3	×	12–15
Crunches	3	×	15–25
Lying Leg Raises	3	×	15–25

Aerobics: 30 minutes; 75% range

DAY #2

Wide Front Pull-downs	4	×	10–12
Barbell Rows	4	×	10–12
Barbell Shrugs	3	×	12–15
Hyperextensions	3	×	20–25
Incline Dumbbell Curls	3	×	12–15
Barbell Curls	4	×	6–8
Two-Dumbbell Wrist Curls	3	×	15–20
Standing Leg Curls	3	×	10–12
Lying Leg Curls	2	×	12–15
Donkey Raises	3	×	8–10
Seated Calf Raises	3	×	15–20

Aerobics: 30 minutes; 75% range

DAY #3
Aerobics: 35-40 minutes; 65-70% range

DAY #4

Incline Flyes	3	×	10–12
Incline Dumbbell Presses	3	×	6–8
▌Dips for Chest	2–3	×	10–12 (bi-set)
▌Across-Bench Pull-overs	2–3	×	15–20 (bi-set)
Upright Rows	3	×	8–10
Alternating Dumbbell Presses	3	×	12–15
Bent-over Side Raises	3	×	8–10
Overhead Pulley Extension	4	×	8–10
Two-Dumbbell Kickbacks	4	×	8–10
Back Squats	3	×	6–8
▌Extension	3	×	15–20 (bi-set)
▌Hack Squats	3	×	15–20 (bi-set)
Hanging Leg Raises	3	×	15–25
Frog Kicks	3	×	15–25

Aerobics: 30 minutes; 75% range

DAY #5

Low-Pulley Rows	4	×	6–8
Wide Rear Pull-downs	4	×	12–15
Half Deadlift/Shrugs	4	×	10–12
Barbell Preacher Curls	4	×	10–12
Concentration Curls	3	×	8–10
Reverse Curl	3	×	12–15
▌Lying Leg Curls	3	×	12–15 (bi-set)
▌Stiff-Leg Deadlifts	3	×	8–10 (bi-set)
Standing Calf Raises	3	×	10–12
Seated Calf Raises	3	×	20–25

Aerobics: 30 minutes; 75% range

DAY #6...#7
No weights or aerobics.

MASTER WEEK 5

DAY #1

Incline Dumbbell Presses	4	×	8–10
Flat Dumbbell Presses	4	×	8–10
Dips for Chest	3	×	10–12
Across-Bench Pull-overs	3	×	15–20
▌Seated Dumbbell Side Raises	3	×	12–15 (bi-set)
▌Presses Behind the Neck	3	×	12–15 (bi-set)
Rear Pulley Crunches	4	×	8–10
Alternating Fronts Dumbbell Raises	3	×	6–8
▌Push-downs	3–4	×	10–12 (tri-set)
▌Bench Dips	3–4	×	10–12 (tri-set)
▌Lying French Presses	3–4	×	10–12 (tri-set)
▌Lying Leg Raises	3	×	15–25 (tri-set)
▌Scissors	3	×	10–12 (tri-set)
▌Twisting Crunches	3	×	15–25 (tri-set)

Aerobics: 30-35 minutes; 70-75% range

DAY #2

Back Squats	4	×	6–8
▌Extensions	3	×	15–20 (tri-set)
▌Hack Squats	3	×	12–15 (tri-set)
▌Sissy Squats	3	×	12–15 (tri-set)
▌Lying Leg Curls	4–5	×	12–15 (bi-set)
▌Stiff-Leg Deadlifts	4–5	×	8–10 (bi-set)
▌Standing Calf Raises	3	×	20–30 (tri-set)
▌Seated Calf Raises	3	×	20–30 (tri-set)
▌Tibia Raises	3	×	20–25 (tri-set)

Aerobics: 30-35 minutes; 75-80% range

DAY #3

Wide Rear Pull-ups	4	×	10–12
Wide Front Pull-downs	3	×	6–8
T-Bar Rows	3	×	8–10
Straight-Arm Pull-ins	3	×	12–15
Barbell Shrugs	4	×	15–20
Hyperextensions	4	×	20–25
Standing Alternating Dumbbell Curls	4	×	10–12
One-arm Preacher Curls	3	×	12–15
Concentration Curls	3	×	6–8
▌Zottman Curls	3	×	12–15 (bi-set)
▌Two-Dumbbell Wrist Curls	3	×	12–15 (bi-set)

Aerobics: 30-35 minutes; 70-75% range

DAY #4

Aerobics: 35-40 minutes; 65-70% range (This is optional. If your body is tired, take a rest from aerobics today.)

DAY #5

Flat Bench Presses	4	×	6–8
▮ Incline Flyes	3	×	10–12 (tri-set)
▮ Incline Dumbbell	3	×	10–12 (tri-set)
▮ Across-Bench Pull-overs	3	×	12–15 (tri-set)
One-Arm Pulley Side Raises	3	×	15–20
Incline Side Raises	3	×	10–12
Bent-over Dumbbell Side Raises	3	×	8–10
Seated Dumbbell Presses	3–4	×	6–8
▮ Push-downs	3	×	10–12 (bi-set)
▮ Two-Dumbbell Kickbacks	3	×	10–12 (bi-set)
▮ Overhead Pulley Extensions	3	×	12–15 (bi-set)
▮ Bench Dips	3	×	8–10 (bi-set)
▮ Hanging Leg Raises	3–4	×	20–25 (tri-set)
▮ Lying Leg Raises	3–4	×	20–25 (tri-set)
▮ Crunches	3–4	×	20–25 (tri-set)

Aerobics: 35 minutes; 75% range

DAY #6

Standing Leg Curls	4	×	15–20
▮ Lying Leg Curls	3	×	8–10 (bi-set)
▮ Stiff-Leg Deadlifts	3	×	12–15 (bi-set)
Leg Extensions	4	×	20–25
Hack Squats	3	×	6–8
45-Degree Leg Presses	3	×	6–8
Standing Calf Raises	4	×	12–15
Donkey Calf Raises	3	×	10–12
Tibia Raises	3	×	15–20

Aerobics: 35 minutes; 75% range

DAY #7

Straight-Arm Pull-ins	4	×	12–15
Barbell Rows	4	×	10–12
Wide Rear Pull-downs	4	×	8–10
Barbell Shrugs	3	×	15–20
Good Mornings	3	×	15–20
Concentration Curls	4	×	12–15
Incline Dumbbell Curls	3	×	8–10
One-Arm Pulley Curls	3	×	8–10
Reverse Curls	3	×	10–12
Two-Dumbbell Wrist Curls	3	×	12–15

Aerobics: 35 minutes; 75% range

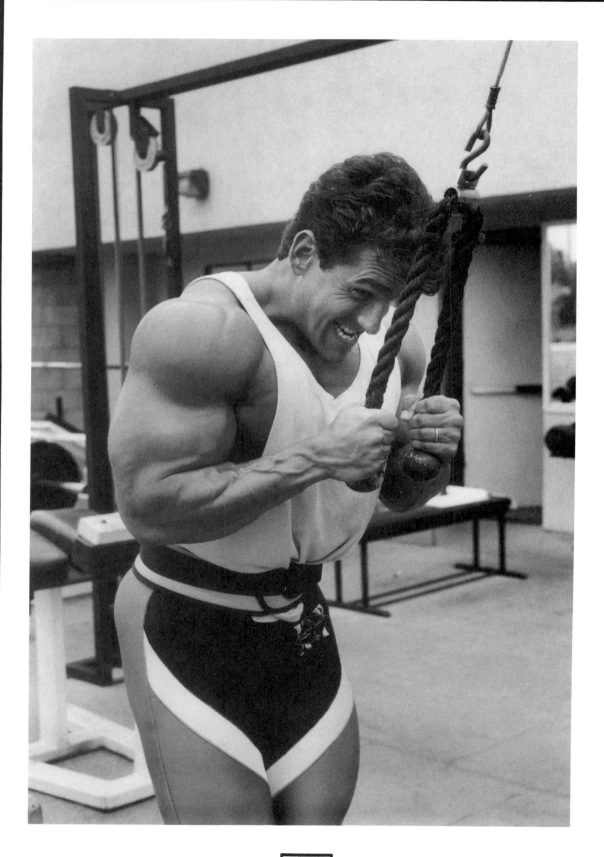

WEEK 6

Well, here you are, just past the halfway point. You should really be seeing and feeling the results of your hard work at this point.

Are you the kind of person who sees the glass of water as half full or half empty? More specifically, do you see yourself having accomplished five weeks of dedication or having five hard weeks to go?

In the purest sense, neither view is perfect. Obviously, an entire volume on human psychology could be written on this subject, and many have been. To keep things simple, I'd like to suggest you find a balance between savoring the accomplishments of the last five weeks and appreciating the work involved in the weeks to come. Don't be too quick to move on from the work you've done, but don't wallow in it at the expense of the task at hand, either.

Let your experiences during the last five weeks serve your next five. In this way you can truly listen to your body and remain enlightened and adaptable to its needs. Obviously, those needs should be judged within the framework of the goal you have set for yourself.

The mind-to-muscle link is much more than just developing nerve pathways that lead to efficient contractions. It's also the link that separates the successful trainer from the rigid, frustrated one.

TRAINING

How sore should a body part get after a workout? There's no way to answer this question simply. However, I personally don't feel that I've trained a body part right unless it's sore for at least a couple of days after training it. I've heard experts say that soreness won't set in for one or two days. But my body parts are usually hurting within a few hours of an intense training session and continue to have a good soreness that slowly intensifies and then diminishes over the course of around three days. My goal is to have the body part fully recovered by its next workout, and one of the ways I gauge that recovery is the ache I feel when I flex it. When the ache is gone, generally the body part is recovered and ready to work again.

Soreness throughout the whole body or sustained muscular aches could be indicators of either overtraining or improper nutrition. These aspects go hand in hand. Your nutrition will help dictate the speed of your muscular recovery and your exercise intensity will dictate your nutritional needs.

You also need to keep your senses keen to separate the good ache from an actual injury or one that may be building. There is a world of difference between that well-worked, fatigued, achy feeling, and chronically hurting connective tissue such as an injured joint, tendon or ligament. You also need to watch for chronically tight muscle fibers that can be precursors of muscle tears. For example, if you use your fingers to explore the muscles of your front deltoid and the pec near where the deltoid and chest tie together, you will probably find what feels like strands of muscle fibers that feel tighter and more tender than the others around them. I point out the pec/deltoid tie-in because it's a frequently injured area for bodybuilders. I had some problems with fiber tightness in my pec/deltoid tie-ins a few years ago and found that intense self-massage in the area helped alleviate some pain and speed up recovery. I would use my fingertips and press them into the tight fibers. I would trace those tight fibers for their whole length (for example, from the front of the armpit up toward the collarbone) and massage them along that entire length to loosen their spasms.

I would also use ice packs on the area immediately following a chest or shoulder workout. I'd keep the ice on the vulnerable area for ten or fifteen minutes and then use my massage technique when the skin returned to its normal temperature. I'd then follow this whole process with a hot bath and be sure my chest/deltoids soaked for ten or fifteen minutes. In the gym I really focused on stretching the pec/deltoid tie-in before and after any upper-body workouts to loosen those fibers. This self-therapy worked for me in a dramatically positive way and can work for any of the areas most vulnerable to overuse or ballistic injuries. Some of those areas are:

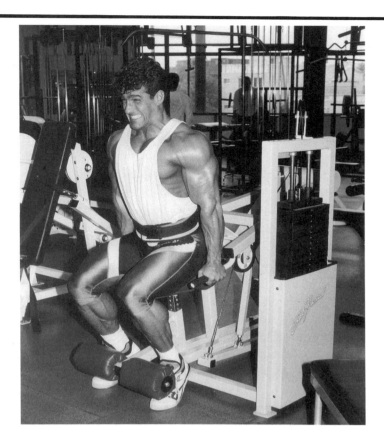

1. **Pec/deltoid tie-in**
2. **Lower biceps tie-in**
3. **Lower triceps tie-in**
4. **Rhomboid/infraspinatus area lying just above the lat muscle and between the rear deltoid and trapezius**
5. **Lower spinal-erector tie-in**
6. **Lower quad/knee area**
7. **Upper forearm/outer biceps tie-in where the elbow bends**
8. **Trapezius/neck tie-in**

There are other areas vulnerable to injury from overly spasmed muscle fibers, but as you can see, the examples above deal exclusively with areas where two body parts merge. These areas tend to get overworked due to overlaps in body part workouts, but a combination of stretching, massage, ice and hot baths can provide positive recuperative benefit. If, however, there is an injury, you must see a doctor. It could mean the difference between a very minor problem and the need for surgery or other invasive techniques. Be smart; being injured and ignoring it will always catch up with you.

NUTRITION

What's all the fuss about medium-chain triglyceride oils—M.C.T.'s? Are they a miracle, fad, fraud or what?

My answer is that although M.C.T.'s have been heralded in some circles as the bodybuilder's miracle supplement, they're just another fad. The addition of M.C.T.'s to the diet *will* help some people reach their goals faster, but it will inhibit others. The people who can benefit from M.C.T. supplementation are in the minority. My conclusion—and it's shared by others who are in a position to know—is that M.C.T.'s best serve those individuals who have such a high metabolism that no amount of clean-food calories can meet their caloric need. If a basic calorie level can't be met, then weight gain is not possible.

It was only after I had a disastrous experience with M.C.T. oil use and began to collect more facts, that I realized M.C.T.'s don't do one single thing to speed up the metabolism or to trigger body-fat loss. Nor do they speed up muscle gain. M.C.T.'s are a fat—simply that. I experimented with using medium to high quantities of M.C.T.'s in my diet for nearly a year. For every day of that period I had stomachaches and a bloated feeling. I also exceeded my caloric needs, making efficient fat loss impossible. The worst thing that happened was that my metabolism slowed down and it took me eighteen months to get it back on track. For me, M.C.T.'s were a nightmare.

Unless you have the metabolism of a hummingbird, I'd recommend staying as far away from M.C.T. oil as possible—especially in large quantities. If you use M.C.T.'s, you must add their calories to your daily fat calorie total. There is no special magic that separates fat calories in M.C.T.'s from fat calories gained via any other source.

JOURNEYMAN WEEK 6

DAY #1

Incline Bench Presses	3	×	6–8
Flat Dumbbell Presses	3	×	10–12
Cable Crossovers on Machine	3	×	15–20
Seated Dumbbell Side Raises	3	×	10–12 (tri-set)
Seated Barbell Presses Behind the Neck	3	×	10–12 (tri-set)
Seated Bent-over Side Raises	3	×	10–12 (tri-set)

Push-downs	4	×	10–12
Bench Dips	4	×	12–20
Hack Squats	3	×	15–20
45-Degree Leg Presses	3	×	12–15
Extensions	3	×	12–15
Crunches	3	×	15–25
Lying Leg Raises	3	×	15–25

Aerobics: 30 minutes; 75% range

DAY #2

Wide Front Pull-downs	4	×	10–12
Barbell Rows	4	×	10–12
Barbell Shrugs	3	×	12–15
Hyperextensions	3	×	20–25
Incline Dumbbell Curls	3	×	12–15
Barbell Curls	4	×	6–8
Two-Dumbbell Wrist Curls	3	×	15–20
Standing Leg Curls	3	×	10–12
Lying Leg Curls	3	×	12–15
Donkey Raises	3	×	8–10
Seated Calf Raises	3	×	15–20

Aerobics: 30 minutes; 75% range

DAY #3

Aerobics: 35-40 minutes; 65-70% range

DAY #4

Incline Flyes	3	×	10–12
Incline Dumbbell Presses	3	×	6–8
▌ Dips for Chest	2–3	×	10–12 (bi-set)
▌ Across-Bench Pull-overs	2–3	×	15–20 (bi-set)
Upright Rows	3	×	8–10
Alternating Dumbbell Presses	3	×	12–15
Bent-over Side Raises	3	×	8–10
Overhead Pulley Extensions	4	×	8–10
Two-Dumbbell Kickbacks	4	×	8–10
Back Squats	3	×	6–8
▌ Leg Extensions	3	×	15–20 (bi-set)
▌ Hack Squats	3	×	15–20 (bi-set)
Hanging Leg Raises	3	×	15–25
Frog Kicks	3	×	15–25

Aerobics: 30 minutes; 75% range

DAY #5

Low-Pulley Rows	4	×	6–8
Wide Rear Pull-downs	4	×	12–15
Half Deadlift/Shrugs	4	×	10–12
Barbell Preacher Curls	4	×	10–12
Concentration Curls	3	×	8–10
Reverse Curls	3	×	12–15
▌Lying Leg Curls	3	×	12–15 (bi-set)
▌Stiff-Leg Deadlifts	3	×	8–10 (bi-set)
Standing Calf Raises	3	×	10–12
Seated Calf Raises	3	×	20–25

Aerobics: 30 minutes; 75% range

DAY #6...#7

No weights or aerobics.

MASTER WEEK 6

DAY #1

Aerobics: 35-40 minutes; 65-70% range (This is optional. If your body is tired, take a rest from aerobics today.)

DAY #2

Incline Dumbbell Presses	4	×	6–8
Incline Dumbbell Presses	4	×	10–12
Flat Flyes	3	×	10–12
Cable Crossovers	3	×	15–20
▌Down-the-Rack Side Raises*	3	×	8–10 (bi-set)
▌Seated Presses Behind the Neck	3	×	10–12 (bi-set)
Two-Pulley Rear Crunches	4	×	12–15
Lying French Presses	4	×	10–12
Rope Push-downs	4	×	12–15
Two-Arm, One-Dumbbell Extensions	3	×	6–8
▌Lying Leg Raises	3–4	×	20–25
▌Frog Kicks	3–4	×	20–25
▌Crunches	3–4	×	20–25

Aerobics: 35 minutes; 75% range

*Three weight drops. In a down-the-rack set, the three tiers combined constitute one set. In this instance, do the three weight tiers and move, in bi-set fashion, to the press.

DAY #3

Extensions	4	×	10–12
Back Squats	4	×	6–8
Lunges	4	×	12–15
Down-the-Rack Lying Legs Curls (Three Weight Drops)	4	×	8–10
Stiff-Leg Deadlifts	3	×	12–15
Leg-Press Calf Raises	4	×	20–25
▎Seated Calf Raises	4	×	15–20 (bi-set)
▎Tibia Raises	4	×	15–20 (bi-set)

Aerobics: 35 minutes; 75% range

DAY #4

Wide Front Pull-ups	4	×	10–12
Wide Front Pull-downs	4	×	12–15
▎Straight-Arm Pull-ins	3	×	8–10 (bi-set)
▎Low-Pulley Rows	3	×	6–8 (bi-set)
Half Deadlift/Shrugs	4	×	10–12
Standing Alternating Dumbbell Curls	4	×	8–10
Barbell Curls	3	×	6–8
One-Dumbbell Preacher Curls	3	×	12–15
Pulley Compound Wrist Curls	3	×	12–15

Aerobics: 35 minutes; 75% range

DAY #5

Aerobics: 35-40 minutes; 65-70% range (This is optional. If your body is tired, take a rest from aerobics today.)

DAY #6

Flat Bench Presses	4	×	6–8
▎Incline Flyes	3	×	10–12 (tri-set)
▎Incline Dumbbell Presses	3	×	10–12 (tri-set)
▎Across-Bench Pull-overs	3	×	12–15 (tri-set)
One-Arm Pulley Side Raises	3	×	15–20
Incline Side Raises	3	×	10–12
Bent-over Dumbbell Side Raises	3	×	8–10
Seated Dumbbell Raises	3–4	×	6–10
▎Push-downs	3	×	10–12 (bi-set)
▎Two-Dumbbell Kickbacks	3	×	10–12 (bi-set)
▎Overhead Pulley Extensions	3	×	12–15 (bi-set)
▎Bench Dips	3	×	8–10 (bi-set)
▎Hanging Leg Raises	3–4	×	20–25 (tri-set)
▎Lying Leg Raises	3–4	×	20–25 (tri-set)
▎Crunches	3–4	×	20–25 (tri-set)

Aerobics: 35 minutes; 75% range

DAY #7

Standing Leg Curls	4	×	15–20
▌Lying Leg Curls	3	×	8–10 (bi-set)
▌Stiff-Leg Deadlifts	3	×	12–15 (bi-set)
Leg Extensions	4	×	20–25
Hack Squats	3	×	6–8
45-Degree Leg Presses	3	×	6–8
Standing Calf Raises	4	×	12–15
Donkey Calf Raises	3	×	10–12
Tibia Raises	3	×	15–20

Aerobics: 35 minutes; 75% range

WEEK 7

No matter what, keep pushing forward. Don't miss workouts; don't skip meals; don't blow off your motivation exercises. Even if you don't feel motivated, go to the gym anyway. Just go in and start your workout. As I've said previously, you might be very surprised at what great training sessions you'll have on days where you just feel like pulling the covers up over your head. Whether the workout is great or mediocre, at least you won't miss it.

I want you to prove something to yourself. Show yourself that you have what it takes to keep going back for more. No one can lift the weights for you. No one but you can find the stuff to push for five more reps on the leg press when your mind is screaming to stop, but your gut knows those quads ain't finished yet.

You are the one who reaches down inside and grabs "it." That elusive "it" is what separates the trainers with warriorlike flawlessness from those who just flap their lips about "someday." Your goal is in sight. Move into high gear and reach for it.

TRAINING

Is it possible to shape a muscle through exercise? This question is causing quite a debate in bodybuilding circles. Those who say that muscle shaping is not possible claim that all an athlete needs are the most basic movements to build mass in body parts, since the actual shape of a body part is enhanced or limited according to genetics.

As you might guess, I disagree with this point of view entirely. Why? Because I continually observe it being disproven. What is muscle shape, anyway? It is the visual illusion presented by a body part, which can be enhanced or destroyed by the strategic development of different sections of the individual muscle.

The anti-shapers theorize that if you only did bench presses for your chest, full development would still take place. I suppose this is possible, but only if you're a genetic freak. For 99.99 percent of athletes, including myself, the bench press is a limited developer that works only one section of a complex body part.

I don't mean to single out the bench press. In fact, the same could be said of dumbbell flyes, dips, barbell curls, triceps push-downs or any of an endless list of exercises. The point is that no single exercise will fully develop any body part. With the chest alone you have four main areas that all need development: the lower, upper, inner and outer chest areas. Then you have even more esoteric subareas, such as inner-lower, outer-upper, etc. Each of those areas requires different angles, hand spacing, and equipment to effectively develop. Therefore, exercise variety is the key to muscle shaping.

What a tragedy if muscle shape was really dictated and fully limited by genetics. I, for one, would have never looked at my own untrained seventeen-year-old body and said, "This kid has really great muscle shapes and will build a symmetrical body."

NUTRITION

What is the greatest factor contributing to the current hardness and leanness of competitive bodybuilders? Some might say drugs, but with the increase in drug testing the sport is definitely more drug-free than it was five or ten years ago.

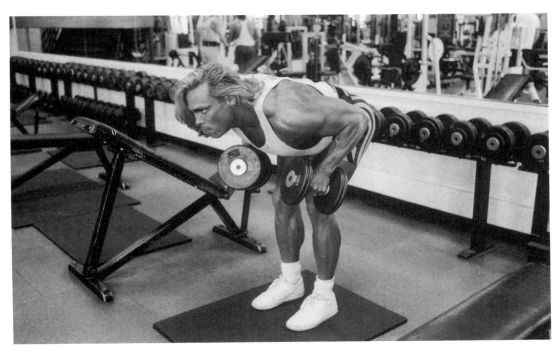

For the triceps to achieve its full potential, it must be worked in a *variety* of different ways—with Dumbbell Kickbacks, for example. The photo above shows the stretch position.

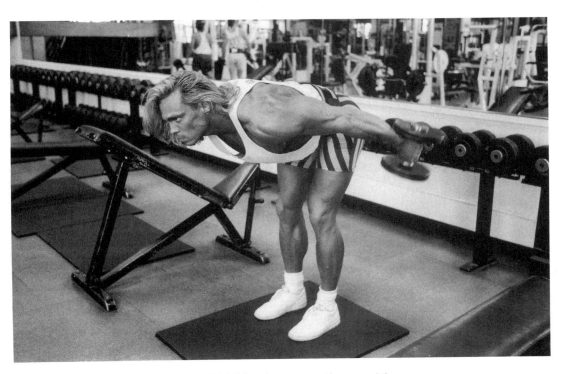

Dumbbell Kickback contraction position.

I think the answer to the leanness-and-hardness question lies in nutrition. The competitive bodybuilder who wants to succeed today must stay in lean condition nearly year-round. If there is one thing I know to be true, it is this: The longer an athlete stays in lean, hard shape, the leaner and harder that athlete becomes. It's a matter of staying in peak condition without burning out. What has evolved for many in the course of this balancing act is a more moderate, longer-range approach. In the past, bodybuilders usually "bulked-up" in the off-season and severely dieted to prepare for a show. What happened to the athlete was very similar to the pattern you see in most crash-diet situations—extreme deprivation followed by binging. With each downward and upward weight swing, the body hoards more fat and becomes more resistant to the next bout of crash dieting.

That is the last thing anyone wants. So intelligent athletes began practicing balanced, clean eating on a year-round basis. In my own case, I may have to drop my calories into the 2,500–3,000 range to get to a low level of body fat, but I can maintain that body-fat level almost indefinitely—assuming my training and recovery remain consistent—by eating 3,500 to 4,500 calories per day. With those additional calories I really begin to see improvements in muscle size and strength. I kind of grow into my peak muscularity.

This is a concept that you should consider during this program and beyond. Work toward your flawless body during these ten weeks and then stay consistent year-round to maximize leanness and hardness.

JOURNEYMAN WEEK 7

DAY #1

Dips for Chest	3	×	12–15 (bi-set)
Low-Incline Flyes	3	×	12–15 (bi-set)
Pec-Decks	3	×	10–12 (bi-set)
Incline Dumbbell Presses	3	×	6–8 (bi-set)
Dumbbell Side Raises	3	×	12–15
Rear Pulley Crunches	3	×	12–15
Barbell Presses Behind the Neck	3	×	6–8
Reverse Push-downs	4	×	10–12
Seated French Presses	4	×	15–20
Back Squats	4	×	8–12
45-Degree Leg Presses	4	×	15–20
Leg Raises	3	×	15–25 (tri-set)
Scissors	3	×	15–25 (tri-set)
Crunches	3	×	15–25 (tri-set)

Aerobics: 30-35 minutes; 75% range

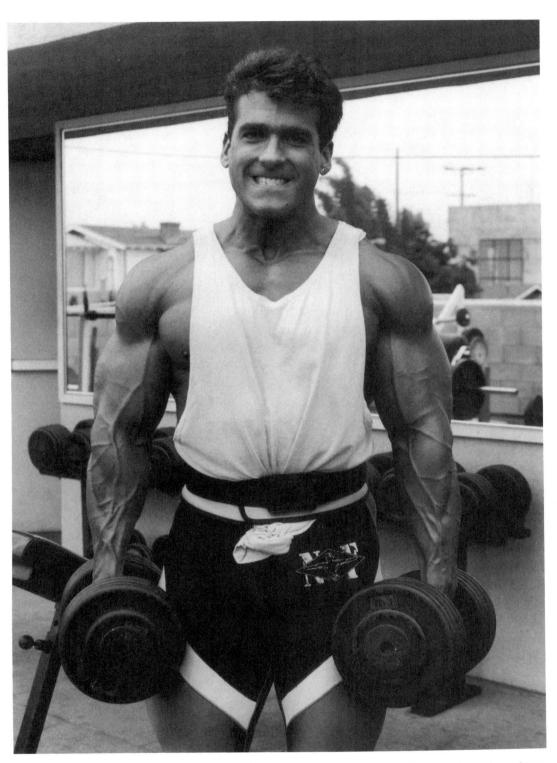

The type of vascularity shown above is achieved by consistently maintaining a low body-fat level.

DAY #2

Wide Front Pull-downs	4	×	10–12
Close-Grip Pull-downs	4	×	8–10
Half Deadlift/Shrugs	3	×	10–12
Hyperextensions	2	×	20–25
Alternating Dumbbell Curls	4	×	6–8
One-Dumbbell Preacher Curls	4	×	12–15
Barbell Wrist Curls	3	×	15–20
Standing Leg Curls	4–5	×	12–20
▌Leg-Press Calf Raises	3	×	12–15 (bi-set)
▌Seated Calf Raises	3	×	12–15 (bi-set)

Aerobics: 30-35 minutes; 75% range

DAY #3

Aerobics: 35-40 minutes; 65-70% range

DAY #4

Flat Bench Presses	3	×	6–8
Incline Bench Presses	3	×	6–8
Incline Flyes	3	×	12–15
Across-Bench Pull-overs	2	×	15–20
One-Arm Pulley Side Raises	3	×	10–12
Incline Side Raises	3	×	10–12
Bent-over Pulley Side Raises	3	×	10–12
▌Push-downs	3	×	12–15 (tri-set)
▌Bench Dips	3	×	10–12 (tri-set)
▌Overhead Pulley Extensions	3	×	10–12 (tri-set)
Leg Extensions	4	×	15–20
Hack Squats	4	×	8–10
Twisting Crunches	5	×	15–25

Aerobics: 30-35 minutes; 75% range

DAY #5

T-Bar Rows	3	×	15–20
One-Dumbbell Rows	3	×	6–8
Wide Front Pull-downs	3	×	6–8
Dumbbell Shrugs	3	×	15–20
Incline Dumbbell Curls	4	×	10–12
Barbell Preacher Curls	3	×	10–12
Reverse Curl	3	×	12–15
Stiff-Leg Deadlifts	3	×	12–15
Lying Leg Curls	4	×	15–20
Standing Calf Raises	3	×	10–12

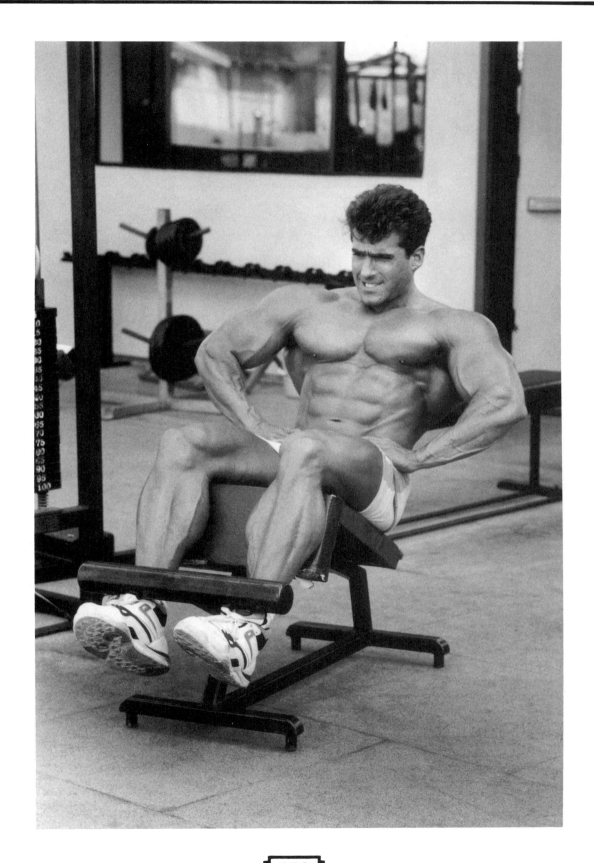

Donkey Raises	3	×	15–20

Aerobics: 30-35 minutes; 75% range

DAY #6...#7

No weights or aerobics.

MASTER WEEK 7

DAY #1

Straight-Arm Pull-ins	4	×	12–15
Barbell Rows	4	×	10–12
Wide Rear Pull-downs	4	×	8–10
Barbell Shrugs	3	×	15–20
Good Mornings	3	×	15–20
Concentration Curls	4	×	12–15
Incline Dumbbell Curls	3	×	8–10
One-Arm Pulley Curls	3	×	8–10
Reverse Curls	3	×	10–12
Two Dumbbell Wrist Curls	3	×	12–15

Aerobics: 35 minutes; 75% range

DAY #2

Aerobics: 35-40 minutes; 65-70% range (This is optional. If your body is tired, take a rest from aerobics today.)

DAY #3

Incline Bench Presses	4	×	6–8
Incline Dumbbell Presses	4	×	10–12
Flat Flyes	3	×	10–12
Cable Crossovers	3	×	15–20
▌Down-the-Rack Side Raises*	3	×	8–10 (bi-set)
▌Seated Presses Behind the Neck	3	×	10–12 (bi-set)
Two-Pulley Rear Crunches	4	×	12–15
Lying French Presses	4	×	10–12
Rope Push-downs	4	×	12–15
Two-Arm, One-Arm Dumbbell			
Extensions	3	×	6–8
▌Lying Leg Raises	3–4	×	20–25 (tri-set)
▌Frog Kicks	3–4	×	20–25 (tri-set)
▌Crunches	3–4	×	20–25 (tri-set)

Aerobics: 35 minutes; 75% range

*Three weight drops. In a down-the-rack set, the three tiers combined constitute one set. In this instance, do the three weight tiers and move, in bi-set fashion, to the press.

DAY #4

Extensions	4	×	10–12
Back Squats	4	×	6–8
Lunges	4	×	12–15
Down-the-Rack Lying Leg			
▌Curls (Three Weight Drops)	4	×	8–10
Stiff-Leg Deadlifts	3	×	12–15
Leg-Press Calf Raises	4	×	20–25
▌Seated Calf Raises	4	×	15–20 (bi-set)
▌Tibia Raises	4	×	15–20 (bi-set)

Aerobics: 35 minutes; 75% range

DAY #5

Wide Rear Pull-downs	4	×	12–15
Low-Pulley Rows	4	×	6–8
One-Dumbbell Rows	4	×	6–8
▌Dumbbell Shrugs	4	×	10–12 (bi-set)
▌Hyperextensions	4	×	10–12 (bi-set)
▌Incline Dumbbell Curls	3	×	8–10 (tri-set)
▌Two-Arm Preacher Curls	3	×	8–10 (tri-set)
▌Two-Arm Pulley Rows	3	×	8–10 (tri-set)
Zottman Curls	3	×	12–15
Barbell Wrist Curls	3	×	15–20

Aerobics: 35 minutes; 75-80% range

DAY #6

Aerobics: 35-40 minutes; 65-70% range (This is optional. If your body is tired, take a rest from aerobics today.)

DAY #7

Flat Dumbbell Presses	4	×	8–10
Incline Dumbbell Presses	4	×	6–8
Pec-Decks	4	×	15–20
Across-Bench Pull-overs	3	×	10–12
Barbell Presses Behind the Neck	3	×	6–8
Upright Rows	3	×	8–10
Incline Side Raises	3	×	8–10
Bent-over Pulley Side Raises	3	×	10–15
Push-downs	4	×	15–20
Barbell Kickbacks	4	×	10–12
One Arm Extensions	4	×	12–15
Hanging Leg Raises	4	×	20–25
Twisting Crunches	4	×	20–25

Aerobics: 35 minutes; 75-80% range

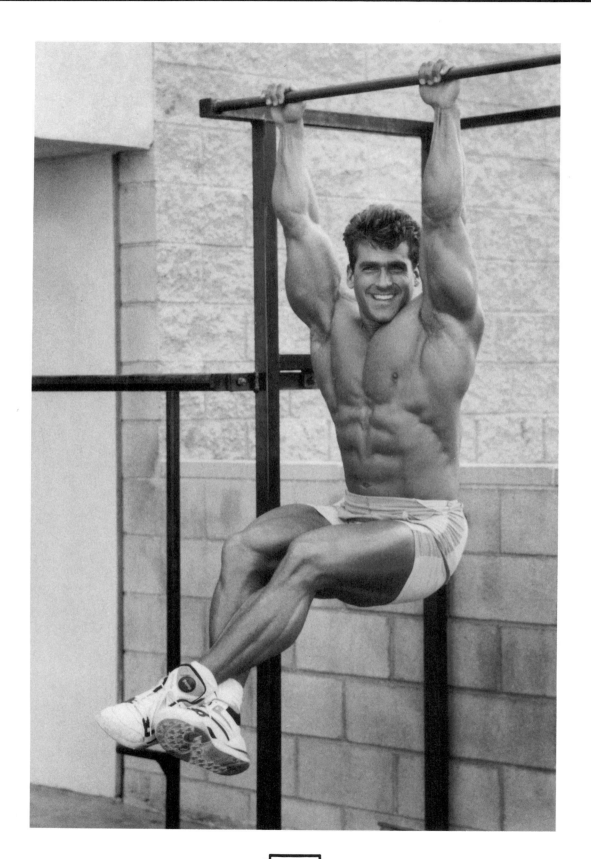

WEEK 8

The end is now in sight. You do, however, still have three weeks of intense work ahead, and you should gear yourself up for this final push.

As you forge onward, try to balance out every aspect of your program. Always listen to your body, so that you'll know the difference between pushing too hard and taking it too easy. Also, as I've said repeatedly, you must navigate the fine line between expectations that are too high and those that are too low.

TRAINING

While I feel that overuse of forced reps (reps taken beyond failure, via the assistance of a partner or by some other method) can hold back a bodybuilder's progress, there are other techniques that, when used moderately and intelligently, can push progress past levels achieved through exclusive use of single-set positive-failure exercises. Those techniques fall under the general heading of compound sets. Remember, though, that compound sets, just like forced reps, are valuable, productive techniques only when they are not abused. What are compound sets?

I see compound sets in two different ways. The first class of compound sets are those that consist of two or more exercises grouped together and performed with no rest in between. In this case, the combined exercises can work either the same or different body parts, and fall under the following guidelines:

Super-set: Combining two different body-part exercises together to form one compound set. Many times super-sets will be done using one exercise each for two opposing muscle groups. For example: biceps and triceps; chest and back; abs and lower back; front thighs and hamstrings.

Using this technique, a biceps exercise would be performed to positive failure. Then you'd move with no rest to a predesignated triceps exercise, and it, too, would be done to positive failure. You'd rest, then repeat the super-set.

There is also a technique I call loose super-setting. You would still use two opposing muscle exercises, but would take a standard rest in between each exercise instead of moving straight from one to the other, then resting.

This technique is beneficial at times when you want a longer rest time for each body part but still want the overall workout to move at a fast pace.

I personally feel more challenged by the standard super-setting technique.

Bi-set, tri-set, giant set: This is when two, three or more exercises for the same body part are done with no rest in between. The rest would come at the end of one compound set. An example of a chest bi-set would be grouping flat flyes with incline dumbbell presses. Do the flyes to positive failure, then move, without rest, to the dumbbell presses. Now rest, catch your breath and start again.

A tri-set would be three exercises done this way, and a giant-set would be four or more. I find four exercise giant-sets to be the desired upper limit. In fact, bi- and tri-sets are the best of this technique, for a couple of reasons. First, most people training in a gym have trouble combining more than two or three exercises, since others also want to use the equipment. The solution is to go to the gym at its most uncrowded time. The second factor involves cardiovascular limitations. If you're going from one exercise to another without rest, you'll get more and more out of breath. So a level needs to be found where you can reach positive failure on each exercise without running out of lung power.

I find that bi-sets and tri-sets are the most underrated advanced technique in bodybuilding. I've seen people achieve dramatic results with intelligent use of these techniques. Once again, they prove the rule that working smart doesn't mean taking it easy.

The second class of compound sets would more accurately be called diminishing sets. There are two types: "down-the-rack" sets and drop sets.

An example of going "down the rack" can be shown with standing dumbbell side raises. You'd start with a weight and do your reps to positive failure. Then you'd set that weight aside and pick up a slightly lighter weight, repping with it to positive failure; set that weight aside and grab a lighter weight, pushing for a third time to positive failure. Then you'd catch your breath and repeat the sequence.

"Down the rack" can be considered a form of self-performed forced reps. This technique must therefore be used cautiously, to allow full recuperation to occur.

Compound-set techniques have been placed at different intervals in your daily training schedules. Use them to your best advantage, but make sure you always allow good recovery for the affected body part. Try stretching, ice after the workout, massage, hot baths and sleep to speed the process.

NUTRITION

Would it hurt you to have an occasional meal or day off from your clean-nutrition plan? "Hurt" is a relative term. It really depends on you, your goal and your level of progress. If you're trying to lose significant weight, then the answer is to stay disciplined.

A wonderful thing happens when you avoid a particular junk food that you crave. Sure, at first your psyche shouts out in protest; it equates the loss of that Twinkie with certain death, or at least extreme discomfort. The wonderful part comes after about four weeks. At that point your craving for this previously addictive food diminishes. Several years ago I found myself in a situation where I was addicted to chocolate-chip cookies. (I had developed this habit when I'd allowed myself to have a few nearly every day just after a contest.) Well, pretty soon I saw that this was becoming destructive. I had another show coming up and I needed to get back on track ASAP.

I went cold turkey. For three weeks I had chocolate on my mind, and then after about four weeks I noticed one day that the craving had just sort of slipped away. I didn't think much about those cookies at all until several weeks later, when I decided to take a "cheat day."

I bought half a dozen of my old favorites, chowed down and then spent the next two weeks fighting the craving again until, once again, it slowly diminished.

If *you* decide to take a "cheat day," don't stuff yourself, and get right back on the clean-eating track the very next day. Your progress will depend on it.

JOURNEYMAN WEEK 8

DAY #1

▌Dips for Chest	3	×	12–15 (bi-set)
▌Low-Incline Flyes	3	×	12–15 (bi-set)
▌Pec-Decks	3	×	10–12 (bi-set)
▌Incline Dumbbell Presses	3	×	6–8 (bi-set)
Dumbbell Side Raises	3	×	12–15
Rear Pulley Crunches	3	×	12–15
Barbell Presses Behind the Neck	3	×	6–8
Reverse Push-downs	4	×	10–12
Seated French Presses	4	×	15–20
Back Squats	4	×	8–12
45-Degree Leg Presses	4	×	15–20
▌Leg Raises	3	×	15–25 (tri-set)
▌Scissors	3	×	15–25 (tri-set)
▌Crunches	3	×	15–25 (tri-set)

Aerobics: 30-35 minutes; 75% range

DAY #2

Wide Front Pull-ups	4	×	10–12
Close-Grip Pull-downs	4	×	8–10
Half Deadlift/Shrugs	3	×	10–12
Hyperextensions	2	×	20–25
Alternating Dumbbell Curls	4	×	6–8
One-Dumbbell Preacher Curls	4	×	12–15
Barbell Wrist Curls	3	×	15–20
Standing Leg Curls	4–5	×	12–20
▌Leg-Press Calf Raises	3	×	12–15 (bi-set)
▌Seated Calf Raises	3	×	12–15 (bi-set)

Aerobics: 30-35 minutes; 75% range

DAY #3

Aerobics: 35-40 minutes; 65-70% range

DAY #4

Flat Bench Presses	3	×	6–8
Incline Bench Presses	3	×	6–8
Incline Flyes	3	×	12–15
Across-Bench Pull-overs	2	×	15–20
One-Arm Pulley Side Raises	3	×	10–12
Incline Side Raises	3	×	12–15
Bent-over Pulley Side Raises	3	×	10–12

Push-downs	3	×	12–15 (tri-set)
Bench Dips	3	×	10–12 (tri-set)
Overhead Pulley Extensions	3	×	10–12 (tri-set)
Leg Extensions	4	×	15–20
Hack Squats	4	×	8–10
Twisting Crunches	5	×	15–25

Aerobics: 30-35 minutes; 75% range

DAY #5

T-Bar Rows	3	×	15–20
One-Dumbbell Rows	3	×	6–8
Wide Front Pull-downs	3	×	6–8
Dumbbell Shrugs	3	×	15–20
Incline Dumbbell Curls	4	×	10–12
Barbell Preacher Curls	3	×	10–12
Reverse Curls	3	×	12–15
Stiff-Leg Deadlifts	3	×	12–15
Lying Leg Curls	4	×	15–20
Standing Calf Raises	3	×	10–12
Donkey Raises	3	×	15–20

Aerobics: 30-35 minutes; 75% range

DAY #6...#7

No weights or aerobics.

MASTER WEEK 8

DAY #1

Front Squats	4	×	6–8
Lunges	3	×	12–15
Hack Squats	4	×	15–20
Standing Leg Curls	4	×	8–10
Lying-Leg Curls	4	×	15–20
Standing Calf Raises	3–4	×	15–20 (tri-set)
Seated Calf Raises	3–4	×	15–20 (tri-set)
Tibia Raises	3–4	×	15–20 (tri-set)

Aerobics: 30 minutes; 75% range

DAY #2

Close-Grip Pull-downs	4	×	10–12
T-Bar Rows	4	×	12–15
Wide-Grip Low-Pulley Rows	4	×	8–10

Half Deadlift/Shrugs	4	×	10–12
Alternating Dumbbell Curls	4	×	10–12
One-Dumbbell Preacher Curls	3	×	10–12
Barbell Curls	3	×	6–8
Pulley Compound Wrist Curl	3	×	12–15

Aerobics: 35 minutes; 75-80% range

DAY #3

Aerobics: 35-40 minutes; 65-70% range (This is optional. If your body is tired, take a rest from aerobics today.)

DAY #4

Incline Flyes	4	×	12–15
Flat Bench Presses	4	×	6–8
Dips	3	×	10–12
Cable Crossovers on Incline Bench	3	×	12–15
Down-the-Rack Side Raises	3	×	12–15
(Three Weight Drops)	3	×	8–10
Down-the-Rack Bent-over Side Raises			
(Three Weight Drops)	3	×	8–10
Lying Compound Side Raises	3	×	12–15
Down-the-Rack Push-downs			
(Three Weight Drops)	3	×	8–10
Lying French Presses	3	×	10–12
Two-Dumbbell Kickbacks	3	×	12–15
▌ Hanging Leg Raises	4–5	×	20–25 (bi-set)
▌ Frog Kicks	4–5	×	20–25 (bi-set)

Aerobics: 35 minutes; 75-80% range

DAY #5

▌ Extensions	3–4	×	15–20 (tri-set)
▌ 45-Degree Leg Presses	3–4	×	20–25 (tri-set)
▌ Sissy Squats	3–4	×	15–20 (tri-set)
▌ Down-the-Rack Lying Leg Curls			
(Three Weight Drops)	3–4	×	8–10 (bi-set)
▌ Stiff-Leg Deadlifts	3–4	×	15–20 (bi-set)
Donkey Calf Raises	4	×	12–15
Seated Calf Raises	4	×	8–10
Tibia Raises	3	×	15–20

Aerobics: 35 minutes; 75-80% range

DAY #6

Wide Rear Pull-downs	4	×	12–15
Low-Pulley Rows	4	×	6–8
One-Dumbbell Rows	4	×	6–8
▌Dumbbell Shrugs	4	×	10–12 (bi-set)
▌Hyperextensions	4	×	20–25 (bi-set)
▌Incline Dumbbell Curls	3	×	8–10 (tri-set)
▌Two-Arm Preacher Curls	3	×	8–10 (tri-set)
▌Two-Arm Pulley Curls	3	×	8–10 (tri-set)
Zottman Curls	3	×	12–15
Barbell Wrist Curls	3	×	15–20

Aerobics: 35 minutes; 75-80% range

DAY #7

Aerobics: 35-40 minutes; 65-70% range (This is optional. If your body is tired, take a rest from aerobics today.)

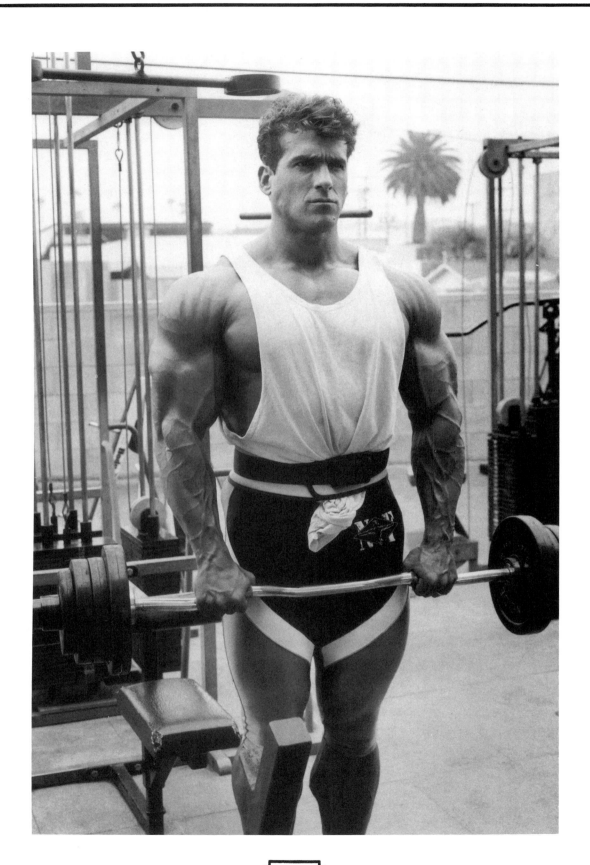

WEEK 9

Do you see your workouts and eating habits as separate from the rest of your life or integrated into it? That's going to be an important question for you to answer as the end of your ten weeks comes into sight.

Are you using this program to meet a short-term goal (e.g., to make an impression at the beach or to dazzle your classmates at your high school reunion) or to put into action positive lifelong habits?

Now, there's nothing wrong with using these ten weeks to get to that goal body; after all, that's what this book is about. However, I hope that during the last eight weeks you've become positively *addicted* to working toward a great physique and all of the positive side effects that go along with that. It's my hope that, even if you started out only wanting to make the greatest possible progress in the shortest amount of time, you began to watch yourself integrate training hard and eating right into the priorities of your life, and as a result felt very good about yourself—good enough to make the flawless lifestyle a permanent one.

TRAINING

There is one major difference between how a bodybuilder should perform any type of deadlifting movement and the way a power lifter performs one. The difference is in the hand grip. A power lifter grips the bar with one palm facing forward and the other facing toward the body. Since a power lifter can't use wrist straps in competition, this grip is used to keep the bar from rolling out of his hands.

For a bodybuilder, though, there's a problem with the alternating hand grip. It concerns the palm that faces forward. By turning the hand in this direction, the biceps is placed in a very vulnerable position, since the hand is in full supination and the biceps is fully stretched. If the stress exerted is too great, the biceps could be strained or torn. Trust me—I've seen it happen more than once, and it's not a pretty sight.

Using different hand grips will also lead to uneven development when doing exercises such as deadlift/shrugs, since every change in hand position causes slightly different direct muscle stimulation. Stick to a dual overhand grip on all deadlifting-type exercises and use wrist straps to physically and psychologically strengthen your grip on the bar.

NUTRITION #1

Let me say this simply—you have no excuse to not consistently eat five or six meals each day. The only way you will make 100 percent progress on this program is by eating all those meals. As long as you can afford to buy the food, nothing should keep you away from your meals. You must become a consistent, disciplined eating machine. If you work away from home or travel, buy several sealable plastic containers, fix and pack all your meals and take them with you. Use a small cooler to keep the food from spoiling.

You must set up an environment for keeping yourself on track. If you think you can wing it at restaurants along the way, you'll be setting yourself up for failure.

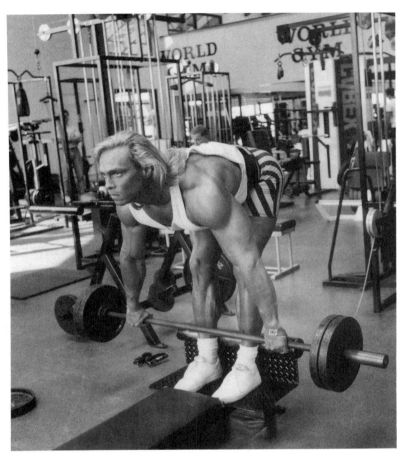

Rod Jackson demonstrates the grip bodybuilders should use in the deadlift movement.

NUTRITION #2

"Eat your vegetables!" You probably haven't heard that phrase since you were a kid. Well, I hate to say this, but now that you're an adult it applies more than ever.

Fibrous vegetables serve as the mortar that holds the bricks of your nutrition together. While protein and complex starchy carbohydrates are the mainstays of a healthy diet, vegetables are the dietary stabilizers. They stabilize your insulin release and therefore your blood sugar. They're also essential in the digestion, assimilation and elimination process that all food goes through. As you'll notice in the nutrition section, every meal after breakfast must include some amount of at least one fibrous vegetable. Hey, you can eat veggies for breakfast, too, if you want! Your basic meal structure should be a protein source, a complex carb source and a fibrous carb source, no matter what your dietary composition percentages are.

JOURNEYMAN WEEK 9

DAY #1

Incline Bench Presses	3	×	8–10
Dips for Chest	3	×	10–12
Cable Crossovers	3	×	12–15
Across-Bench Pull-overs	2	×	15–20
Barbell Presses Behind the Neck	3	×	6–8
Upright Rows	3	×	6–8
Incline Side Raises	3	×	10–12
Lying French Presses	4	×	6–8
Rope Extensions	4	×	10–12
Back Squats	4	×	15–20
Hack Squats	4	×	15–20
▌Hanging Leg Raises	3	×	15–25 (tri-set)
▌Crunches	3	×	15–25 (tri-set)
▌Frog Kicks	3	×	15–25 (tri-set)

Aerobics: 30 minutes; 75% range

DAY #2

Wide Rear Pull-ups	3	×	10–12
Barbell Rows	3	×	8–10
Close-Grip Pull-downs	3	×	15–20
Barbell Shrugs	3	×	10–12
One-Dumbbell Preacher Curls	4	×	12–15
Concentration Curls	3	×	10–12
Standing Leg Curls	4	×	10–12
Stiff-Leg Deadlifts	3	×	12–15
Standing Calf Raises	3	×	15–20
Seated Calf Raises	3	×	8–10

Aerobics: 35 minutes; 75% range

DAY #3

Aerobics: 35-40 minutes; 65-70% range

DAY #4

▌Incline Flyes	3	×	10–12 (bi-set)
▌Incline Dumbbell Presses	3	×	10–12 (bi-set)
Flat Bench Presses	3	×	6–10
▌Seated Bent-over Side Raises	3	×	12–15 (tri-set)
▌Dumbbell Presses	3	×	12–15 (tri-set)
▌Dumbbell Side Raises	3	×	8–10 (tri-set)
▌Push-downs	3–4	×	12–15 (bi-set)
▌Bench Dips	3–4	×	12–15 (bi-set)
▌Leg Extensions	4	×	10–12 (bi-set)
▌45-Degree Leg Presses	4	×	10–12 (bi-set)
Crunches	3	×	20–25
Lying Leg Raises	3	×	20–25

Aerobics: 35 minutes; 75% range

DAY #5

Wide Front Pull-downs	3	×	15–20
Low-Pulley Rows	3	×	12–15
One-Dumbbell Rows	3	×	8–10
Half Deadlift/Shrugs	3	×	10–12
Barbell Curls	4	×	8–10
Incline Dumbbell Curls	3	×	6–8
Reverse Curls	3	×	12–15
Standing Leg Curls	3	×	10–12
Lying Leg Curls	3	×	12–15
Donkey Calf Raises	3	×	8–10
Leg-Press Calf Raises	3	×	10–12

Aerobics: 35 minutes; 75% range

DAY #6...#7

No weights or aerobics.

MASTER WEEK 9

DAY #1

Flat Dumbbell Presses	4	×	8–10
Incline Dumbbell Presses	4	×	6–8
Pec-Decks	4	×	15–20
Across-Bench Pull-overs	3	×	10–12
Barbell Presses Behind the Neck	3	×	6–8
Upright Rows	3	×	8–10
Incline Side Raises	3	×	8–10

Bent-over Pulley Side Raises	3	×	10–15
Push-downs	4	×	15–20
Barbell Kickbacks	4	×	10–12
One-Arm Extensions	4	×	12–15
Hanging Leg Raises	4	×	20–25
Twisting Crunches	4	×	20–25

Aerobics: 30-35 minutes; 75-80% range

DAY #2

Front Squats	4	×	6–8
Lunges	3	×	12–15
Hack Squats	4	×	15–20
Back Squats	4	×	15–20
Standing Leg Curls	4	×	8–10
Lying-Leg Curls	4	×	15–20
Standing Calf Raises	3–4	×	15–20 (tri-set)
Seated Calf Raises	3–4	×	15–20 (tri-set)
Tibia Raises	3–4	×	15–20 (tri-set)

Aerobics: 30-35 minutes; 75-80% range

DAY #3

Close-Grip Pull-downs	4	×	10–12
T-Bar Rows	4	×	12–15
Wide-Grip Low-Pulley Rows	4	×	8–10
Half Deadlift/Shrugs	4	×	10–12
Alternating Dumbbell Curls	4	×	10–12
One-Dumbbell Preacher Curls	3	×	10–12
Barbell Curls	3	×	6–8
Pulley Compound Wrist Curl	3	×	12–15

Aerobics: 30-35 minutes; 75-80% range

DAY #4

Aerobics: 35-40 minutes; 65-70% range (This is optional. If your body is tired, take a rest from aerobics today.)

DAY #5

Incline Flyes	4	×	12–15
Flat Bench Presses	4	×	6–8
Dips	3	×	10–12
Cable Crossovers on Incline Bench	3	×	12–15
Down-the-Rack Side Raises (Three Weight Drops)	3	×	8–10
Down-the-Rack Bent-over Side Raises (Three Weight Drops)	3	×	8–10

Lying Compound Side Raises	3	×	12–15	
Down-the-Rack Push-downs (Three Weight Drops)	3	×	8–10	
Lying French Presses	3	×	10–12	
Two-Dumbbell Kickbacks	3	×	12–15	
▌ Hanging Leg Raises	4–5	×	20–25	(bi-set)
▌ Frog Kicks	4–5	×	20–25	(bi-set)

Aerobics: 35 minutes; 75-80% range

DAY #6

▌ Leg Extensions	3–4	×	15–20	(tri-set)
▌ 45-Degree Leg Presses	3–4	×	15–20	(tri-set)
▌ Sissy Squats	3–4	×	15–20	(tri-set)
▌ Down-the-Rack Lying Leg Curls (Three Weight Drops)	3–4	×	8–10	(bi-set)
▌ Stiff-Leg Deadlifts	3–4	×	15–20	(bi-set)
Donkey Calf Raises	4	×	12–15	
Seated Calf Raises	4	×	8–10	
Tibia Raises	3	×	15–20	

Aerobics: 35 minutes; 75-80% range

DAY #7

▌ Straight-Arm Pull-ins	3–4	×	12–15	(tri-set)
▌ Wide Front Pull-downs	3–4	×	12–15	(tri-set)
▌ Two-Dumbbell Rows	3–4	×	12–15	(tri-set)
Dumbbell Shrugs	4	×	15–20	
Hyperextensions	4	×	20–25	
One-Arm Pulley Curls	4	×	10–12	
One-Dumbbell Preacher Curls	4	×	12–15	
Concentration Curls	3	×	6–8	
▌ Zottman Curls	3	×	12–15	(bi-set)
▌ Two-Dumbbell Wrist Curls	3	×	12–15	(bi-set)

Aerobics: 35 minutes; 75-80% range

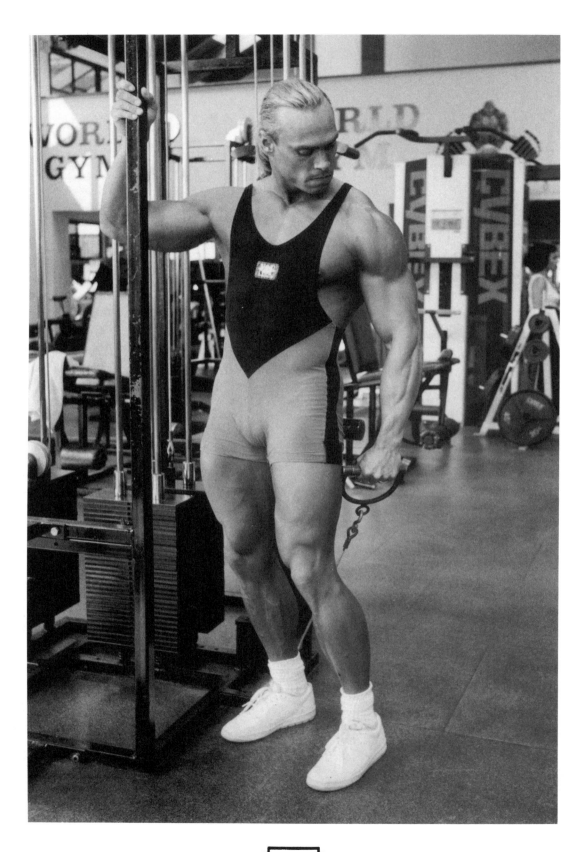

WEEK 10

Welcome to Week 10. After all your hard work, you should be very proud of yourself. When I sat down to write this introduction to the final week of the program, I realized something: Aside from the new tips included here, there is basically nothing I can say to you at this point that I haven't already said.

You know how to focus in. You know how to feel the muscles. You know how to eat and how to recover from the workouts. You also know how to visualize your perfect body, how to motivate yourself to train hard and eat right and how to put all those elements together to fit your needs.

You're one week from accomplishing your goal. Congratulations! It's been great working together.

TRAINING #1

I could never imagine avoiding squats in my workouts, and they were especially important during those years when I was building the foundation of my physique. But many people do shun them, for a lot of different reasons. I think squats are mostly avoided because they're a hard, intense exercise involving great muscular, cardiovascular and mental exertion.

The major problem I see people having when they do squats is keeping the front thigh isolated and the butt out of the movement as much as possible. Once again, you should differentiate between how someone lifting for power would squat and the way someone wanting to sculpt massive thighs would. The person lifting purely for power is not interested in such esoterics as muscle isolation. Getting the weight from point A to point B is what is essential, and the more muscle tendons and leverage adding to the effort, the better.

The intelligent bodybuilder doesn't want to build a big butt. In fact, I can't remember anyone requesting a program specializing in building massive glutes. Because of the compound nature of squatting, the glute muscles will always be a secondary muscle worked. The performance of the exercises dictates how great that secondary effect will be.

I keep my front thighs isolated by placing a one-inch block underneath my heels and keeping my feet no more than twelve inches apart. The farther you lean forward during the reps, the more the glutes and lower back become involved, so I focus my eyes upward. I find a place on the wall or ceiling that I have to look up to see when standing straight at the top of the exercise. Throughout the whole range of motion, I keep my visual attention focused on this spot. Looking upward keeps my body upright and the effort focused on the quads. With front squats, of course, there is a greater quad isolation, since leaning forward will mean dumping the bar onto the floor in front of you.

Focus on making your squatting exercises more than just grunt-and-groan efforts. With attention to performance details, they can add mass, isolate and sculpt exactly as you want.

TRAINING #2

You can stretch your way past a stubborn body-part plateau. If training by itself isn't helping to bring a lagging body part up to speed, try stretching the muscle between sets on the exercises.

This technique is especially helpful in tight muscles where you feel physical hardness when you do self-massage. Your goal should be a visually hard-looking body, but you should be able to sink your fingers deeply into even the most highly developed muscle group.

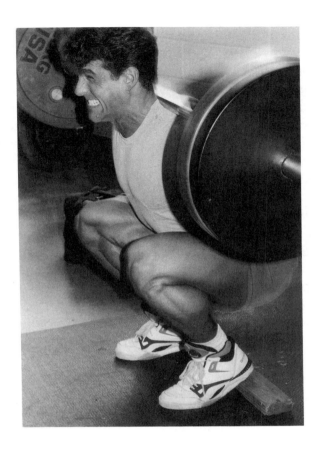

Use the isolating stretch that best fits the body part you are targeting and at the conclusion of each set for that body part stretch the muscle. Do long, slow stretches and hold them for fifteen to twenty seconds without any bouncing. This stretching can also be combined with iso-tension (flexing the muscle) between sets. I've seen this technique really help bring around a stubborn body part when coordinated with an intelligent variety of exercises and reps.

NUTRITION

I learned long ago never to assume that a person understood what I meant when I used the term "clean eating." I recall one instance where a man to whom I'd given a weight-loss diet couldn't lose weight. His training was consistent, and when I asked him about it he claimed he was following my nutritional guidelines. After three months of nonexistent progress, I said to him, "Okay, enough. Tell me exactly what you're eating."

He described all the foods I'd suggested for him. Everything sounded fine, but after some additional prying on my part, I got a valuable insight. It seems some miscommunication had occurred: He didn't understand that having a baked potato meant *just* the potato. He revealed to me, all the while thinking he'd done nothing out of the ordinary, that he was adding about 3,000 calories of extra junk to his food every day. Between butter and sour cream on potatoes, butter in rice, bleu cheese dressing on salads and veggies, brown sugar in his oatmeal and so on, he had completely missed the point of the weight-loss formula.

The solution is to write down in your journal every single bite of food that enters your mouth, remembering that every calorie counts. Now this may seem obvious to you, but it certainly isn't to most.

If you want to perk up your diet, use things like onions, garlic, cinnamon and other spices that add flavor without calories.

Low-fat, low-sodium Mexican salsa also offers flavor without significant calories, but make sure to enter whatever calories it does add into your daily total.

Cooking "clean" means preparing food as close to its natural state as possible. Meat should be grilled, broiled, baked or steamed. Carbs should be prepared without adding fat, and vegetables should be lightly steamed to retain their vitamins and minerals. Don't add oil or butter to anything.

JOURNEYMAN WEEK 10

DAY #1

Incline Bench Presses	3	×	8–10
Dips for Chest	3	×	10–12
Cable Crossovers	3	×	12–15
Across-Bench Pull-overs	2	×	15–20
Barbell Presses Behind the Neck	3	×	6–8
Upright Rows	3	×	6–8
Incline Side Raises	3	×	10–12
Lying French Presses	4	×	6–8
Rope Extensions	4	×	10–12
Back Squats	4	×	15–20
Hack Squats	4	×	15–20
▌ Hanging Leg Raises	3	×	15–25 (tri-set)
Crunches	3	×	15–25 (tri-set)
▌ Frog Kicks	3	×	15–25 (tri-set)

Aerobics: 35 minutes; 75% range

DAY #2

Wide Rear Pull-ups	3	×	10–12
Barbell Rows	3	×	8–10
Close-Grip Pull-downs	3	×	15–20
Barbell Shrugs	3	×	10–12
One-Dumbbell Preacher Curls	4	×	12–15
Concentration Curls	3	×	10–12
Two-Dumbbell Wrist Curls	3	×	15–20
Standing Leg Curls	4	×	10–12
Stiff-Leg Deadlifts	3	×	12–15
Standing Calf Raises	3	×	15–20
Seated Calf Raises	3	×	8–10

Aerobics: 35 minutes; 75% range

DAY #3

Aerobics: 35-40 minutes; 65-70% range

DAY #4

▌ Incline Flyes	3	×	10–12 (bi-set)
▌ Incline Dumbbell Presses	3	×	10–12 (bi-set)
Flat Bench Presses	3	×	10–12
▌ Seated Bent-over Side Raises	3	×	12–15 (bi-set)
▌ Dumbbell Presses	3	×	12–15 (bi-set)
Dumbbell Side Raises	3	×	8–10

▌Push-downs	3–4	×	12–15 (bi-set)
▌Bench Dips	3–4	×	12–15 (bi-set)
▌Leg Extensions	4	×	10–12 (bi-set)
▌45-Degree Leg Presses	4	×	10–12 (bi-set)
Crunches	3	×	20–25
Lying Leg Raises	3	×	20–25

Aerobics: 35 minutes; 75% range

DAY #5

Wide Front Pull-downs	3	×	15–20
Low-Pulley Rows	3	×	12–15
One-Dumbbell Rows	3	×	8–10
Half Deadlift/Shrugs	3	×	10–12
Barbell Curls	4	×	8–10
Incline Dumbbell Curls	3	×	6–8
Reverse Curls	3	×	12–15
Standing Leg Curls	3	×	10–12
Lying Leg Curls	3	×	12–15
Donkey Calf Raises	3	×	8–10
Leg Press Calf Raises	3	×	10–12

Aerobics: 35 minutes; 75% range

DAY #6...#7

No weights or aerobics.

MASTER WEEK 10

DAY #1

Aerobics: 35-40 minutes; 65-70% range (This is optional. If your body is tired, take a rest from aerobics today.)

DAY #2

Dips	4	×	10–12
Incline Bench Presses	4	×	6–8
Incline Flyes	3	×	12–15
Across-Bench Pull-overs	3	×	15–20
Dumbbell Presses	4	×	6–8
▌Two-Pulley Rear Crunches	3–4	×	10–12 (bi-set)
▌Upright Rows	3–4	×	10–12 (bi-set)
One-Arm Push-downs	4	×	12–15
Seated French Presses	3	×	10–12
Bench Dips	4	×	8–10

Lying Leg Raises	3–4	×	20–25 (tri-set)
Frog Kicks	3–4	×	20–25 (tri-set)
Twisting Crunches	3–4	×	20–25 (tri-set)

Aerobics: 35 minutes; 75-80% range

DAY #3

Lying Leg Curls	4	×	10–12
Standing Leg Curls	4	×	10–12
Back Squats	4	×	6–8
Hack Squats	4	×	6–8
Extensions	3	×	15–20
Standing Calf Raises	4	×	15–20
Leg-Press Calf Raises	4	×	6–8
Tibia Raises	3	×	15–20

Aerobics: 35 minutes; 75-80% range

DAY #4

Wide Front Pull-ups	4	×	10–12
Wide Front Pull-downs	4	×	12–15
Standing Alternating Dumbbell Curls	4	×	8–10
Barbell Curls	3	×	6–8
One-Dumbbell Preacher Curls	3	×	12–15
Pulley Compound Wrist Curl	3	×	12–15

Aerobics: 35 minutes; 75% range

DAY #5

Aerobics: 35-40 minutes; 65-70% range (This is optional. If your body is tired, take a rest from aerobics today.)

DAY #6

Flat Bench Presses	4	×	6–8
Incline Flyes	3	×	10–12 (tri-set)
Incline Dumbbell Presses	3	×	10–12 (tri-set)
Across-Bench Pullovers	3	×	10–12 (tri-set)
One-Arm Pulley Side Raises	3	×	15–20
Incline Side Raises	3	×	10–12
Bent-Over Dumbbell Side Raises	3	×	8–10
Seated Dumbbell Presses	3–4	×	6–10
Push-downs	3	×	10–12 (bi-set)
Two-Dumbbell Kickbacks	3	×	10–12 (bi-set)
Overhead Pulley Extensions	3	×	12–15 (bi-set)
Bench Dips	3	×	8–10 (bi-set)

▌ Hanging Leg Raises	3–4	×	20–25 (tri-set)
▌ Lying Leg Raises	3–4	×	20–25 (tri-set)
▌ Crunches	3–4	×	20–25 (tri-set)

Aerobics: 35 minutes; 75% range

DAY #7

Standing Leg Curls	4	×	15–20
▌ Lying Leg Curls	3	×	8–10 (bi-set)
▌ Stiff-Leg Deadlifts	3	×	12–15 (bi-set)
Leg Extensions	4	×	20–25
Hack Squats	3	×	6–8
45-Degree Leg Presses	3	×	6–8
Standing Calf Raises	4	×	12–15
Donkey Calf Raises	3	×	10–12
Tibia Raises	3	×	15–20

Aerobics: 35 minutes; 75% range

Appendix

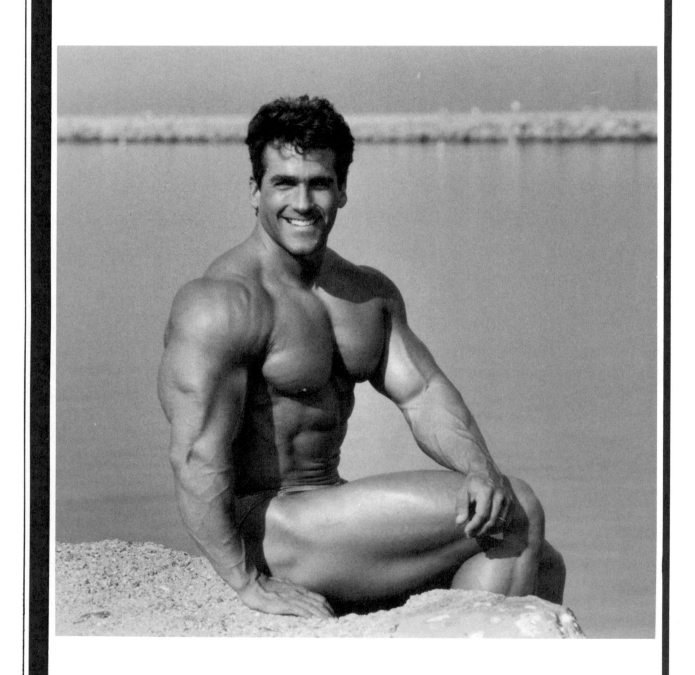

EATING RIGHT

If your two biggest goals in life are creating a flawless body and deciding whose bacon double-cheeseburger is really the best, you've got a problem. The problem is conflicting goals. You've got to sit down and decide what you really want.

Right now I want you to decide exactly what you expect from your nutrition plan over the course of your ten-week program. Do you want to lose weight, gain weight or stay about the same?

It's important to understand that muscle tissue weighs more than fat. Theoretically you could gain weight even if your goal is weight loss by developing larger muscle fibers but reducing fat cells. Most people have a goal of gaining muscle and losing fat simultaneously, no matter what level of experience they have in the gym. In fact, one of the most frequently asked questions at my fitness seminars is how to successfully achieve this change.

It's very much a balancing act. You must eat enough calories to feed your lean-body mass while not consuming more than you will burn during the course of a day. If you consume more calories than your body can use, it will store them as fat. It's like some sort of strange, twisted savings account; in effect, you're storing those extra calories for a rainy day. You see, your body is in many respects a survival mechanism. Accordingly, it constantly makes metabolic adjustments, somewhat like the thermostat on a furnace. It makes the automatic assumption that you might not eat again for a few days or weeks, so it stores extra calories as fat, which can later be recruited to provide energy. This storage business really kicks in if you sharply drop your calories, as in the case of a crash diet. When calories drop, your body responds by slowing down its metabolism so it can survive. Dramatic calorie reduction signals the brain that starvation could be imminent.

The body slows down and doles these calories out very frugally. Little does the body know that it is frustrating its owner by keeping itself fat while being fed half a grapefruit and a lettuce leaf per day. This is why crash dieting does not work.

There is also another factor to consider. Lean-body mass metabolizes calories more efficiently than fat does. The leaner your body is, the higher number of calories it will utilize. A person with a high percentage of body fat will not be able to eat as many calories as a person with low body fat. Although this sounds like some sort of cosmic injustice (kind of like the rich getting richer), it can in fact save someone's life. We know that many health problems go hand in hand with being overweight. The way you eat and the way in which you resolve a high body-fat percentage will likely determine the direction of your health well into the future. Look at a high level of external body fat as an indicator that all might not go smoothly inside the body. Fat doesn't stop at the surface, it pours into the arteries and heart valves.

A word about that term "fat"—as in "overweight." Here, it's not meant as a put-down, just reality. Let's define what is and what isn't "high" body fat. Body fat is "high" when it makes you physically, mentally or emotionally uncomfortable enough to want to change. It should never be confused with an anorexic's or obsessive's excuse for self-flagellation. Every body has fat. Some fat is necessary for normal bodily function. You'll recall that I stated earlier in the book that your goal should be lowering your body fat to a level that you can maintain on a daily basis without starvation. If you've got a little bit of a love handle hanging over the elastic on your underpants, that doesn't make you obese. But, if you put your nose to the grindstone and get to work, you can get your fat down to its lowest maintainable point and keep it there.

HOW TO EAT

The basics of nutrition are that if you want to gain weight you eat more calories during the course of a day than you burn, and if you want to lose weight you eat fewer calories than you actually use during a day. The complicated part comes in how your body responds to different types of calories.

There used to be a popular theory that it didn't matter if you ate 500 calories of chicken breast or 500 calories of tapioca pudding, your body would see both sets of calories the same. This theory looks great on paper, but in reality it is completely false.

My personal experience is that all other things being equal (workout duration, aerobics, recuperation), my body will respond and function at least 100 times better on 4,000 clean calories (lean protein, complex carbohydrates and low fat) than on 4,000 junk-food calories (high fat and simple carbohydrates, e.g., sugar).

Your body will always function better if your daily calories come from clean, wholesome foods, prepared as close to their natural state as possible. Think about it. All that butter, lard, mayonnaise, french fries and candy going down your throat is like pouring a bucket of mud into your bathroom sink and expecting the drain to work right.

The bottom line: If you want a flawless body, you must eat *clean*. Eating clean means:

1. **Fresh lean meat**
2. **Complex carbohydrates**
3. **Fresh vegetables**
4. **Fresh fruit**
5. **Nonfat dairy products**
6. **The low-fat portion of eggs (white)**

Eating clean doesn't mean:

1. **Butter or its substitutes on anything**
2. **Foods with a fat content higher than 10 percent**
3. **Deep-fried anything**
4. **Salad dressing or mayonnaise**
5. **Any food that is high in fat, sugar or salt**

When you eat clean, how should your calories be broken down? What percentage of calories should be protein, carbohydrates and fats?

The standard for balanced diets at the moment seems to be 20 to 25 percent protein, 60 to 65 percent carbohydrates and 10 to 20 percent fats. This is a terrific nutrition strategy and one that works very well for many people. Yet, there's something I've learned over the years that defies the logic of the balanced-diet dogma.

Some people's bodies just respond better if the percentage of protein calories in the diet is increased. Rather than invoking the old mythology that you have to eat muscle in order to gain muscle, I'm pointing out a metabolic consideration. A lot of athletes have what I call a "protein metabolism." I happen to be one of those people, so this strikes a personal note.

Instead of being scientific, let me explain by personal example. But first let me say that in life I think we go through cycles in our knowledge. We return to things that work but have no explanation, when those things that do have an elaborate, logical explanation fail.

Around 1982 I began to experiment with my nutrition, using what I call "diet cycles." I noticed that I just looked better at times when my protein intake was fairly high. I also realized that I needed to replenish my glycogen stores with carbohydrates, in order to provide fuel for intense workouts and recuperation.

What would happen if I manipulated my calories so that some days were very high in protein, some were high in carbs and some were in a more traditional balance?

With manipulation and experimentation, a pattern developed. The cycles began to follow a weekly pattern. I've incorporated this pattern into one of the diet plans in this section. Basically your nutrition strategy will fall into one of the following two categories:

1. Balanced Nutrition Strategy
2. Diet Cycle Strategy

Which one is right for you? It depends on certain factors that should be carefully considered before deciding. It's vital to understand that no matter which nutrition strategy you use for your ten-week program, the Balanced Nutrition Strategy is the best and healthiest year-round core plan. The Diet Cycle Strategy is not intended to be used all year long; it's most effective for short, goal-oriented time periods. The Diet Cycle Strategy should be viewed as a system that helps some people "jump-start" the process of physical change. In the case of an athlete using this program who's determined that he wants to go with the Diet Cycle Strategy, he'd use that strategy only for the ten weeks of his program. The athlete would then return to a balanced eating plan for the remainder of the year, or until another flawlessness program was initiated. Most find that after ten weeks of cycle dieting, gains can be well maintained using the Balanced Nutrition Strategy.

The *Balanced Nutrition Strategy* should be used by those who:

1. Have less than one year of experience with "clean" nutrition. You must know how your body responds to this core routine first before using more esoteric nutrition plans.

2. Have any health considerations dealing with hypoglycemia, hyperglycemia or diabetes. A balanced diet must be followed if you have any problems with your blood sugar fluctuation levels. You must consult your doctor to make this determination.

3. Have a medium to fast metabolism and naturally moderate to low surface body-fat levels during times of consistent exercise and good nutrition.

4. Have as their primary goal for this program a desire to dramatically improve their eating style. For example, those who want to make a change away from severe overeating or undereating to healthy, balanced nutrition.

5. Have responded positively to balanced nutrition in the past. It should be noted that the majority of weight-training athletes, from recreational to competitive, respond best to this nutrition style. Don't think that the Balanced Nutrition Strategy is for the beginner and the Diet Cycle Strategy is for the advanced. Most pro bodybuilders use balanced dieting in both off-season and precontest periods, with extraordinary success.

The *Diet Cycle Strategy* should be used by those who:

1. Have more than one year of experience with clean, balanced nutrition.

2. Feel that balanced nutrition does not fully lead them to a peak condition and are looking for a jump-start method to break through to that level.

3. Have no problem with severe blood sugar fluctuations as long as meals are spaced evenly throughout the day.

4. Have a medium to slow metabolism.

Given the above criteria, it's up to you to decide which strategy best suits the needs of your individual ten-week program.

CALORIC AVERAGING

The one element that will be consistent in both nutritional strategies is the concept of caloric averaging. It's the nutritional equivalent of my weight-training "variety rule," wherein exercises and repetitions are constantly changed to avoid allowing the body to reach a point of stasis. If your body receives the same number of calories per day on an endless basis, it will grow accustomed to this level and your metabolism will gradually shut down. It's far better to stagger your calorie levels throughout the week in order to confuse the metabolism and keep it working at an efficient level. So some days will have lower or higher calories than others. Let's look at an example week, using 3,000 calories as our goal average:

Day	Calories Per Day
Day 1	2,600
Day 2	3,200
Day 3	2,900
Day 4	3,800
Day 5	2,200
Day 6	3,300
Day 7	3,000

21,000 Total
Week's Calories

21,000 divided by 7 = 3,000 Average Daily Calories.

You should keep this up-and-down pattern going as you plan your daily calories throughout your program. With the Balanced Nutrition Strategy the pattern should be fairly random, as shown in the above example. With the Diet Cycle Strategy there is more of a structure to the pattern, as you'll see.

Since this book is being read by people with a broad range of metabolisms and nutrition goals, I've tried to present plans that as much as possible meet all these needs, without being so generic as to be useless. Each plan is built around a basic calorie level, but also includes caloric options that can be added or taken away.

HOW TO USE THIS SECTION

The information that follows may appear complicated. Don't be intimidated. What appears complex is actually a simplification that will make your nutrition strategy easier, more convenient and more effective.

The first thing you'll encounter in this section is a clean-food list. This is a compilation of the basic foods that you'll be eating over the course of your ten-week program. There are four categories in this section.

1. **Protein foods**
2. **Starchy complex carbohydrate foods**
3. **Vegetables**
4. **Fruits**

Next to each of the foods listed is information about its level of calories, protein, carbohydrates and fats. The numbers given show the values for one ounce (except where otherwise noted).

From this list you can calculate the nutrient values for any food, in any amount, by multiplying the listed figures by the number of ounces you desire.

Say, for example, you want to know the calorie, protein, carbohydrate and fat amounts in eight ounces of red snapper. Simply multiply all the figures across the red snapper line by eight and you'll have your answer.

Why is this important? Because your meal sizes will vary according to the number of total calories you want to consume each day. This clean-food list will be invaluable for your ten-week program and is an extraordinarily useful resource for your future nutrition plans.

Clean-food list with small incremental component breakdowns. All figures are for one ounce of food except where otherwise noted.

PROTEIN SOURCES	CALORIES	PROTEIN	CARBOHYDRATES	FATS
Chicken breast[1]	35	7	0	0.6
Turkey breast[1]	35	7	0	0.6
Flank or round steak[2]	40	6.5	0	1.4
Cod[3]	23	5.3	0	0.1
Red snapper[3]	28	6	0	0.3
Scallops[3]	24	4.6	0	0.1
Whole egg (1 large)	80	6	0.6	5.6
Egg white (1 large)	16	3.4	.41	0
Nonfat milk	10	1	1.4	0.1
Plain nonfat yogurt[4]	13.75	1.5	2.1	0

COMPLEX STARCHY

CARBOHYDRATES	CALORIES	PROTEIN	CARBOHYDRATES	FATS
Oats (dry)	117	4.2	20.4	2.2
Rice (dry wt.)	108	2	24	0.1
Potatoes[5]	22.8	0.6	5.1	0
Sweet Potatoes[5]	34.2	0.5	8	0.1
Lima Beans	30	1.8	5.8	0
Corn	28	1	6.5	0.3
Peas	22	1.6	3.8	0.1

FIBROUS

VEGETABLES[6]	CALORIES	PROTEIN	CARBOHYDRATES	FATS
Asparagus	7.8	.75	1.1	0
Broccoli	9.6	1.1	1.8	0
Brussels sprouts	13	1.4	2.5	0.1
Carrots	12	0.3	2.9	0
Cauliflower	8	1	1.5	0
Cucumbers	4.5	0.2	1	0
Green Beans	9.6	0.6	2.1	0
Lettuce	3.9	0.25	1	0
Mushrooms	8.4	0.8	1.3	0.1
Spinach	7.8	1	1.3	0.1
Zucchini	5.1	0.3	1	0

FRUIT	CALORIES	PROTEIN	CARBOHYDRATES	FATS
Apple	16	.05	4	0.5
Banana	17.5	0.2	4.45	0.1
Blueberries	16	0.2	4	0.1
Cantaloupe	5.7	0.1	1.4	0
Grapefruit	4.5	0.1	1.1	0
Kiwi	15.3	0.25	3.8	0.1
Orange	9.5	0.2	2.4	0
Pear	15.3	0.1	3.8	0.1
Strawberries	8.6	0.2	2	0.1

Footnotes for Calorie List

(1) Skinless and boneless. Weight indicates lean meat only.
(2) All visible fat meticulously removed. Meat finely ground in food processor and drained after cooking.
(3) Broiled, steamed, grilled or poached with *no* added fat.
(4) Plain; no fruit or sweetener added.
(5) Fresh; baked, boiled or steamed only.
(6) Statistics for fresh or frozen with no additives.

BALANCED NUTRITION STRATEGY

I decided on a slightly different approach when creating the next section. It would have been the easiest, but at the same time least effective, thing for me to have written one generic balanced diet for every reader to follow.

That would have been incredibly irresponsible on my part, since every person reading this book has different caloric needs. Instead I've given you the components of your diet, along with illustrating examples.

First is a chart giving the calories necessary in each nutrient category (protein, carbohydrate and fat) broken down according to the traditional balance guidelines of 20 to 25 percent protein, 60 to 65 percent carbohydrates and 10 to 20 percent fats. These breakdowns are given for diets of 2,000, 3,500 and 5,000 calories.

Below that chart is another that gives the same information broken down into increments of 100, 200 and 400 calories. This is done so that you can make day-to-day changes in your caloric level and still know what ranges you're working with.

For example, if you desire a 2,400-calorie day and need to know how many calories come from protein, carbs and fat to stay balanced, you'd simply add the figure for each individual component on the 2,000-calorie chart to the corresponding number on the 400-calorie chart, etc. For a 7,000-calorie day, you would add the component numbers (in the same desired percentage range) from the 5,000- and 2,000-calorie charts.

Before you blow a head gasket worrying that you'll have to do endless calculations to come up with your daily meals, read on. Following these two charts, you'll find that I've done much of the planning and math homework for you.

SAMPLE CALORIES IN BALANCED PROPORTIONS

	PERCENT	2,000 CALORIES	3,500 CALORIES	5,000 CALORIES
Protein	20	400	700	1,000
	25	500	875	1,250
Carbohydrates	60	1,200	2,100	3,000
	65	1,300	2,275	3,250
Fats	10	200	350	500
	15	300	535	750
	20	400	700	1,000

CALORIE EXAMPLES IN 100- , 200- and 400-CALORIE UNITS WITH CORRECT BALANCED PROPORTION RANGES

	PERCENT	100 CALORIES	200 CALORIES	400 CALORIES
Protein	20	20	40	80
	25	25	50	100
Carbohydrates	60	60	120	240
	65	65	130	260
Fats	10	10	20	40
	15	15	30	60
	20	20	40	80

THE MEALS

Using the food chart listed earlier, combined with the percentage ranges necessary to keep a balanced, clean eating plan, I developed the following sample meals. Each meal is in either a 400- , 600- or 800-calorie category. Each meal contains:

1. **The foods that will be eaten**
2. **The exact portion of each food**
3. **The number of calories provided by that portion**
4. **The grams of protein**
5. **The grams of carbohydrates**
6. **The grams of fat**
7. **The totals for the meal**

I've tried as much as possible to stay in the traditional balanced ranges, but sometimes go slightly over or under on one component or another. It's the closeness to the desired range that's the goal—even if it's not exact.

Four sample menus are given in each of the 400- , 600- and 800-calorie meal plans. You'll also notice that I have broken down the 400- and 600-calorie meals even further. To give you flexibility and easy knowledge in moving individual meal calories up or down, 100-calorie breakdowns are provided for all meals (please note that the 400- and 800-calorie charts are the same meals). If you want to turn the 400-calorie Meal #4 into 500 calories, simply add the portions listed for each food from the 100-calorie Meal #4 chart and you'll have your 500 calories.

Use an accurate food scale to weigh your food and get your portions as close as possible. Remember, the more you invest in this program, the more you'll get out of it.

400-CALORIE MEALS IN TRADITIONAL BALANCE

400-CALORIE MEAL #1

Food	Quantity	Calories	Protein	Carbs	Fat
Round steak	2.25 ounces	90	14.7	0	3.2
Lima beans	2.75 ounces	82.5	5	16	0
Rice	2.0 ounces	216	4	48	0.2
Spinach	1.5 ounces	11.7	1.5	2	0.2
		400.2	2.52	66.0	3.6

400-CALORIE MEAL #2

Food	Quantity	Calories	Protein	Carbs	Fat
Whole Egg	½ egg	40	3	0.3	2.8
Egg whites	3.5	56	12	1.45	0
Oatmeal	2 ounces	234	8.4	40.8	4.4
Nonfat Milk	2 ounces	20	2	2.8	0.2
Banana	3 ounces	52.5	0.6	13.4	0.3
		402.5	26	58.75	7.7

400-CALORIE MEAL #3

Food	Quantity	Calories	Protein	Carbs	Fat
Turkey breast	2.5 ounces	87.5	17.5	0	1.5
Corn	5 ounces	140	5	32.5	1.5
Peas	5 ounces	110	8	19	0.5
Brussels sprouts	5 ounces	65	7	12.5	0.5
		402.5	37.5	64	4.0

400-CALORIE MEAL #4

Food	Quantity	Calories	Protein	Carbs	Fat
Scallops	1.5 ounces	36	6.9	0	0.15
Flank steak	1.5 ounces	60	9.75	0	2.1
Sweet potato	7.5 ounces	256.5	3.75	60	0.75
Cauliflower	3 ounces	24	3	4.5	0
Zucchini	5 ounces	25.5	1.5	5.0	0
		402	24.9	69.5	3.0

100-CALORIE INCREMENTS FOR 400-CALORIE TRADITIONAL BALANCED MEALS

MEAL #1

Food	Quantity
Round steak	0.6 ounces
Lima beans	0.7 ounces
Rice	0.5 ounces
Spinach	0.4 ounces

MEAL #2

Food	Quantity
Whole egg	⅛ yolk
Egg white	1 white
Oatmeal	0.5 ounces
Nonfat milk	0.5 ounces
Banana	0.75 ounces

MEAL #3

Food	Quantity
Turkey breast	0.6 ounces
Corn	1.25 ounces
Peas	1.25 ounces
Brussels sprouts	1.25 ounces

MEAL #4

Food	Quantity
Scallops	0.4 ounces
Flank steak	0.4 ounces
Sweet potato	2.0 ounces
Cauliflower	0.75 ounces
Zucchini	1.0 ounces

600-CALORIE MEALS IN TRADITIONAL BALANCE

600-CALORIE MEAL #1

Food	Quantity	Calories	Protein	Carbs	Fat
Egg whites	5	80	17	2	0
Oatmeal	4 ounces	468	16.8	81.6	8.8
Strawberries	2 ounces	17.2	0.4	4	0.4
Nonfat Milk	4 ounces	40	4	5.6	0.4
		605.2	38.2	93.2	9.6

600-CALORIE MEAL #2

Food	Quantity	Calories	Protein	Carbs	Fat
Flank steak	4 ounces	160	26	0	12.6
Sweet potato	10 ounces	342	6	51	0
Corn	3 ounces	84	3	19.5	1.0
Broccoli	2 ounces	19	2.2	3.6	0
		605	37.2	74.1	13.6

600-CALORIE MEAL #3

Food	Quantity	Calories	Protein	Carbs	Fat
Chicken breast	6 ounces	210	42	0	3.6
Rice	3.5 ounces	378	7.0	84	0.4
Green beans	2 ounces	19.2	1.2	4.1	0
		607.2	50.2	88.1	4.0

600-CALORIE MEAL #4

Food	Quantity	Calories	Protein	Carbs	Fat
Cod	3.5 ounces	80.5	18.6	0	0.35
Baked potato	15 ounces	342	9	76.5	0
Whole eggs	2	160	12	1.2	11.2
Asparagus	3 ounces	23.4	2.2	3.3	0
		605.9	41.8	81.0	11.55

100-CALORIE INCREMENTS FOR 600-CALORIE TRADITIONAL BALANCED MEALS

Meal #1

Food	Quantity
Egg white	1 ounce
Oatmeal	0.6 ounces
Strawberries	0.3 ounces
Nonfat Milk	0.6 ounces

Meal #2

Food	Quantity
Flank steak	0.7 ounces
Sweet potato	1.7 ounces
Corn	0.5 ounces
Broccoli	0.3 ounces

Meal #3

Food	Quantity
Chicken breast	7.0 ounces
Rice	0.6 ounces
Green beans	0.3 ounces

Meal #4

Food	Quantity
Cod	0.6 ounces
Baked potato	2.5 ounces
Whole egg	1/3 whole egg
Asparagus	0.5 ounces

800-CALORIE MEALS IN TRADITIONAL BALANCED MEALS

800-Calorie Meal #1

Food	Quantity	Calories	Protein	Carbs	Fat
Round steak	4.5 ounces	180	29.3	0	6.3
Lima beans	5.5 ounces	165	10	32	0
Rice	4 ounces	432	8	96	0.4
Spinach	3 ounces	23.4	3	4	0.4
		800.4	50.3	132	7.1

800-CALORIE MEAL #2

Food	Quantity	Calories	Protein	Carbs	Fat
Whole eggs	1	80	6.0	0.6	5.6
Egg whites	7	112	24	2.9	0
Oatmeal	4 ounces	468	16.8	81.6	8.8
Nonfat milk	4 ounces	40	4	5.6	0.4
Banana	6 ounces	105	1.2	26.7	0.6
		805	52	117.4	15.4

800-CALORIE MEAL #3

Food	Quantity	Calories	Protein	Carbs	Fat
Turkey breast	5 ounces	175	35	0	3
Corn	10 ounces	280	10	65	3
Peas	10 ounces	220	16	38	1
Brussels sprouts	10 ounces	130	14	25	1
		805	75	128	8.0

800-CALORIE MEAL #4

Food	Quantity	Calories	Protein	Carbs	Fat
Scallops	3 ounces	72	13.8	0	0.3
Flank steak	3 ounces	120	19.5	0	4.2
Sweet potato	15 ounces	513	7.5	120	1.5
Cauliflower	6 ounces	48	6	9	0
Zucchini	10 ounces	51	3.0	10.0	0
		804	49.8	139	6.0

WHERE TO GO FROM HERE

Your next step is to determine how many calories you want to average per day. This is an area where I can give you some rough guidelines, but not a specific answer. You must use your best judgment in determining your individual calorie level, according to your goals and needs. One thing to keep in mind is that with this program and all the variable components I've made available, you can adjust your average calorie level from week to week in order to move closer to your goal.

What if your goal is weight loss and you decide to begin at 3,000 calories? After two weeks you may be seeing good effects from your training, but not noticing a drop in body fat. In such a case, your caloric level is probably too high.

I'd solve that by dropping the average daily calories to 2,500 for the next two weeks and monitoring your progress when consuming that amount of food.

The converse is also true. If your goal is weight gain and 3,000 calories is not working, move the level up to 4,000 and remain open to making adjustments throughout the ten weeks. What you need is a starting point, a reasonable calorie level where you can begin. Above all else, be flexible. If one level isn't working, make an adjustment.

If you're trying to lose weight and are disciplined, dedicated and flexible, it's reasonable (and healthy) to expect a weight loss of one to four pounds per week averaged over your ten-week program. But that will most likely fluctuate from week to week. It's much more difficult to pin down figures for weight gain. Most people could wash down five dozen doughnuts a day with two gallons of rocky road ice cream and expect to gain vast amounts of bodyweight over ten weeks. Gaining muscle, on the other hand, is a much more difficult process. For most, muscular weight gains come in much smaller increments than gains in fat.

A hardworking intermediate-level bodybuilder who is committed to building muscle size can usually gain four to seven pounds of pure muscle per year. An advanced, pro-level bodybuilder's increases will probably be much smaller—one to four pounds per year of solid muscle. Put the emphasis on "the look" instead of the sheer numbers.

Here are *rough* guidelines for determining individual caloric starting points. I leave it up to you to decide if you have a slow, medium or fast metabolism.

Slow Metabolism

A. Goal of quality weight loss: 1,700–2,000 calories.
B. Goal of quality weight gain: 2,500–3,500 calories.

Medium Metabolism

A. Goal of quality weight loss: 2,000–2,500 calories.
B. Goal of quality weight gain: 3,000–4,000 calories.

Fast Metabolism

A. Goal of quality weight loss: 2,500–3,500 calories.
B. Goal of quality weight gain: 3,500–7,000 calories.

Your meals should be divided into as many as you can possibly schedule through the day. Eating five or six meals (while staying in your calorie range) is the most effective approach. The minimum number should be four.

The high number of meals will keep your body fed regularly throughout the day and prevent dramatic blood sugar fluctuations.

It will also keep you from overstuffing your stomach at each feeding. Your digestion will be much more effective with six small meals than with three big ones.

If you're on a low-calorie program and you eat six meals each day, the relative meal size may be small; those six small meals will still keep your cravings to a minimum.

I would strongly suggest, by the way, that you invest in a small food scale. This way you will know how much eight ounces of chicken breast really is. Use your journal to record every bite of food that goes into your mouth. Be honest—if in order to maintain a false image you add or delete food you've eaten, you'll only stall your progress.

REVIEW OF NUTRITIONAL GUIDELINES

1. Determine the average calorie range that best suits your body type and goal.

2. Familiarize yourself with the calorie breakdown charts.

3. Develop an up-and-down calorie level for each day of the week that will average out to your desired calorie amount.

4. Break each day into increments of four to six meals. Start the day with high-calorie meals and work downward.

5. Use either the preplanned meals or create balanced meals using the calorie guide.

6. Weigh all food before preparation. Stay with recommended guidelines.

7. Prepare in advance all meals to be eaten away from home. Be prepared and you can avoid rationalizations and excuses for breaking your routine.

8. Record in your journal all food consumed so that you can best know the effect you are creating.

DIET CYCLE STRATEGY

The way this strategy works is that every day of the week you cycle not only your caloric levels, but also your percentages of protein, carbohydrates and fats.

In a sense what you're doing with this approach is nutritionally depleting the muscle of glycogen and then refilling it on a continuous cycle. I personally experience an increase (or at least stabilization and no decrease) in lean-muscle mass and a dramatic decrease in body fat over the course of several weeks using this system.

The following charts and meals come from my own journal notes, taken over years of experience and system refinement.

You should be aware that on your low-calorie, low-carbohydrate days (Days 1, 2, 3, and 7), your energy levels may suffer slightly. Mental concentration levels may also be slightly lower on these days. You are depleting the fuel source (glycogen) that stokes your muscles and brain. So a *slight* "spaciness" and lethargy may be experienced. If it is dramatic, your overall calories may be too low.

In the gym, you may also find that positive failure is reached quicker, but on higher-calorie carbohydrate days the exact opposite will be true. The nature of the cycle is to deplete and load.

Once again, please note that this program can have its difficult moments and is definitely not for everyone. All I can tell you is this—if it works for you, you will swear by it. Analyze your progress on a week-to-week basis. If you aren't getting the results you want from this strategy, first check to ensure you are following the pattern correctly and that your training and recuperation are in order.

You can switch strategies at any point in your ten-week flawlessness program. Remember to be flexible, but also be persistent and determined. The program should really be failing before you make the switch.

THE CYCLES

What follows is information taken from my journals to give you an idea of the day-to-day nature of this system. You'll notice that calorie averaging is still being used here, but in a set pattern. In the following example, 3,000 calories are my desired daily average.

This chart lists daily calories; percentage breakdown of protein, carbs and fat; and the percentage of 3,000 calories that each day's total calories represent.

DAILY CALORIES	PERCENT OF AVERAGE DAILY CALORIES	PERCENT OF PROTEIN	PERCENT OF CARBS	PERCENT OF FATS
		DAY 1		
1,900	64	65	25	10
		DAY 2		
2,400	80	65	20	15
		DAY 3		
3,000	100	55	35	10
		DAY 4		
3,200	106	45	40	15
		DAY 5		
4,200	140	35	50	15
		DAY 6		
3,700	123	25	65	10
		DAY 7		
2,600	87	55	35	10

The percentage of the daily average is provided to enable you to determine your daily caloric level, no matter if your average weekly calories are 2,000 or 8,000. Multiply your average number of calories by the indicated percentage to determine your daily level.

The next two charts are similar to ones used in the balanced nutrition section. The first gives caloric breakdowns for 2,000- , 3,500- and 5,000-calorie diets in the correct daily ratios specific to the cycle diet. The second does the same thing in 100- , 200- and 400-calorie increments. These charts, combined with the earlier clean-food lists, are valuable references in creating your daily menus.

DIET CYCLE STRATEGY SAMPLE CALORIE BREAKDOWNS

DAY 1

COMPONENT	PERCENTAGE	2,000	3,500	5,000
Protein	65	1,300	2,275	3,250
Carbs	25	500	875	1,250
Fat	10	200	350	500

DAY 2

COMPONENT	PERCENTAGE	2,000	3,500	5,000
Protein	65	1,300	2,275	3,250
Carbs	20	400	700	1,000
Fat	15	300	525	750

DAY 3

COMPONENT	PERCENTAGE	2,000	3,500	5,000
Protein	55	1,100	1,925	2,750
Carbs	35	700	1,225	1,750
Fat	10	200	350	500

DAY 4

COMPONENT	PERCENTAGE	2,000	3,500	5,000
Protein	45	900	1,575	2,250
Carbs	40	800	1,400	2,000
Fats	15	300	525	750

DAY 5

COMPONENT	PERCENTAGE	2,000	3,500	5,000
Protein	35	700	1,225	1,750
Carbs	50	1,000	1,750	1,750
Fat	15	300	525	750

DAY 6

COMPONENT	PERCENTAGE	2,000	3,500	5,000
Protein	25	500	875	1,000
Carbs	65	1,300	2,275	3,250
Fat	10	200	350	500

DAY 7

COMPONENT	PERCENTAGE	2,000	3,500	5,000
Protein	55	1,100	1,925	2,750
Carbs	35	700	1,225	1,750
Fat	10	200	350	500

DIET CYCLE STRATEGY SAMPLE CALORIES BROKEN DOWN INTO
100- , 200- and 400-CALORIE INCREMENTS

DAY 1

COMPONENT	PERCENTAGE	100	200	400
Protein	65	65	130	260
Carbs	25	25	50	100
Fat	10	10	20	40

DAY 2

COMPONENT	PERCENTAGE	100	200	400
Protein	65	65	130	260
Carbs	20	20	40	80
Fat	15	15	30	60

DAY 3

COMPONENT	PERCENTAGE	100	200	400
Protein	55	55	110	220
Carbs	35	35	70	140
Fat	10	10	20	40

DAY 4

COMPONENT	PERCENTAGE	100	200	400
Protein	45	45	90	180
Carbs	40	40	80	160
Fat	15	15	30	60

DAY 5

COMPONENT	PERCENTAGE	100	200	400
Protein	35	35	70	140
Carbs	50	50	100	200
Fat	15	15	30	60

DAY 6

COMPONENT	PERCENTAGE	100	200	400
Protein	25	25	50	100
Carbs	65	65	130	260
Fat	10	10	20	40

DAY 7

COMPONENT	PERCENTAGE	100	200	400
Protein	55	55	110	220
Carbs	35	35	70	140
Fat	10	10	20	40

Here is a seven-day diet cycle sample based on my own journals and taken from a 3,000-calorie-per-day average.

1,900 CALORIES; APPROXIMATELY 65% PROTEIN, 25% CARBS, 10% FAT

DAY 1

MEAL #1

Food	Quantity	Calories	Protein	Carbs	Fat
Egg whites	14	224	47.6	1.4	0
Turkey breast	3.5 ounces	122.5	24.5	0	2.1
Oatmeal	1 ounce	117	4.2	20.4	2.2
Strawberries	4 ounces	34.4	0.8	8.0	0.4
		497.9	77.1	29.8	4.7

MEAL #2

Food	Quantity	Calories	Protein	Carbs	Fat
Red snapper	9 ounces	252	54	0	2.7
Egg whites	10 ounces	160	34	4.1	0
Spinach	6 ounces	46.8	6	7.8	0.6
		458.8	94	11.9	3.3

MEAL #3

Food	Quantity	Calories	Protein	Carbs	Fat
Chicken breast	8 ounces	280	56	0	4.8
Lima beans	3.5 ounces	105	6.3	20.3	0
Brussels sprouts	3 ounces	39	4.8	7.5	0.8
		424	67.1	27.8	5.6

MEAL #4

Food	Quantity	Calories	Protein	Carbs	Fat
Flank steak	7 ounces	280	45.5	0	9.8
Baked potato	4 ounces	91.2	2.4	20.4	0
Carrots	2 ounces	24	0.6	5.8	0
		395.2	48.5	26.2	9.8

MEAL #5 (Postworkout)

Food	Quantity	Calories	Protein	Carbs	Fat
Sweet Potato	4.5 ounces	154	2.3	36	0.5

2,400 CALORIES; APPROXIMATELY 65% PROTEIN, 20% CARBS, 15% FAT

DAY 2

MEAL #1

Food	Quantity	Calories	Protein	Carbs	Fat
Egg whites	11	176	37.4	4.5	0
Flank steak	9 ounces	360	58.5	0	12.6
Oatmeal	1 ounce	117	4.2	20.4	2.2
		653	100.1	24.9	14.8

MEAL #2

Food	Quantity	Calories	Protein	Carbs	Fat
Chicken breast	16 ounces	560	112	0	9.6
Broccoli	4 ounces	38.4	4.4	7.2	0
		598.4	116.4	7.2	9.6

MEAL #3

Food	Quantity	Calories	Protein	Carbs	Fat
Round steak	11 ounces	440	71.5	0	15.4
Corn	3 ounces	84	3	19.5	0.9
Cauliflower	3 ounces	24	3	4.5	0
		548	77.5	24.0	16.3

MEAL #4

Food	Quantity	Calories	Protein	Carbs	Fat
Scallops	13 ounces	312	59.8	0	1.3
Zucchini	3 ounces	15.3	0.9	3.0	0
		327.3	60.7	3.0	1.3

MEAL #5 (Postworkout)

Food	Quantity	Calories	Protein	Carbs	Fat
Rice	2.5 ounces	270	5	60	0.25

3,000 CALORIES; APPROXIMATELY 55% PROTEIN, 35% CARBS, 10% FAT

DAY 3

MEAL #1

Food	Quantity	Calories	Protein	Carbs	Fat
Egg whites	12	192	40.8	5	0
Turkey breast	10 ounces	350	70.0	0	6.0
Oatmeal	1 ounce	117	4.2	20.4	2.2
Sweet potato	4 ounces	137	2.0	32.0	0.4
		796	117	57.4	8.6

MEAL #2

Food	Quantity	Calories	Protein	Carbs	Fat
Chicken breast	16 ounces	560	112	0	9.6
Rice	1 ounce	108	2	24	0.1
Broccoli	4 ounces	38.4	4.4	7.2	0
		706.4	118.4	31.2	9.7

MEAL #3

Food	Quantity	Calories	Protein	Carbs	Fat
Turkey breast	9 ounces	315	63	0	5.6
Lima beans	6 ounces	180	10.8	34.8	0
Peas	5 ounces	132	8	19	0.5
Spinach	3 ounces	23.4	3	3.9	0.3
		650.4	84.8	57.7	6.4

MEAL #4

Food	Quantity	Calories	Protein	Carbs	Fat
Red snapper	12 ounces	336	72	0	3.6
Rice	1.5 ounces	162	3	36	0.15
Green beans	6 ounces	57.6	3.6	12.6	0
		555.6	78.6	48.6	3.75

MEAL #5

Food	Quantity	Calories	Protein	Carbs	Fat
Sweet potato	8.5 ounces	290	4.25	68	0.85

3,200 CALORIES; APPROXIMATELY 45% PROTEIN, 40% CARBS, 15% FAT

DAY 4

MEAL #1

Food	Quantity	Calories	Protein	Carbs	Fat
Egg whites	10	160	34	4.1	0
Flank steak	8 ounces	320	52	0	11.2
Oatmeal	3 ounces	351	12.6	61.2	6.6
Banana	4 ounces	70	0.8	17.8	0.4
		901	99.4	83.1	18.2

MEAL #2

Food	Quantity	Calories	Protein	Carbs	Fat
Egg whites	12	192	40.8	5.0	0
Turkey breast	7 ounces	245	49	0	4.2
Oatmeal	2 ounces	234	8.4	40.8	4.4
Sweet potato	4 ounces	137	2.0	32.0	0.4
		808	100.2	77.8	9.0

MEAL #3

Food	Quantity	Calories	Protein	Carbs	Fat
Chicken breast	10 ounces	350	70	0	6
Rice	3 ounces	324	6	72	0.3
Broccoli	4 ounces	38.4	4.4	7.2	0
		712.4	80.4	79.2	6.3

MEAL #4

Food	Quantity	Calories	Protein	Carbs	Fat
Red snapper	12 ounces	336	72	0	3.6
Rice	1 ounce	108	2	24	0.1
Green beans	6 ounces	57.6	3.6	12.6	0
		501.6	77.6	36.6	3.7

MEAL #5 (Postworkout)

Food	Quantity	Calories	Protein	Carbs	Fat
Sweet Potato	8.5 ounces	290	4.25	68	0.85

4,200 CALORIES; APPROXIMATELY 35% PROTEIN, 50% CARBS, 15% FAT

DAY 5

MEAL #1

Food	Quantity	Calories	Protein	Carbs	Fat
Whole eggs	3	240	18	1.8	16.8
Egg whites	6	96	20.4	2.5	0
Oatmeal	3 ounces	351	12.6	61.2	6.6
Banana	4.5 ounces	75	0.9	20	0.45
Nonfat milk	4 ounces	40	0	0	0
		802	51.9	85.5	23.85

MEAL #2

Food	Quantity	Calories	Protein	Carbs	Fat
Turkey breast	5 ounces	175	35	0	3.0
Corn	10 ounces	280	10	65	3.0
Peas	10 ounces	220	16	38	1.0
Brussels sprouts	10 ounces	130	14	25	1.0
		805	75	128	8.0

MEAL #3

Food	Quantity	Calories	Protein	Carbs	Fat
Cod	4.7 ounces	108	25	0	0.5
Whole eggs	3	240	18	1.8	16.8
Baked potato	20 ounces	456	12	102	0
Asparagus	4 ounces	31	3	4.4	0
		835	58	108.2	17.3

MEAL #4

Food	Quantity	Calories	Protein	Carbs	Fat
Flank steak	5.5 ounces	220	35.75	0	7.7
Sweet potato	13.5 ounces	462	6.75	108	1.35
Corn	4 ounces	112	4	26	1.2
Broccoli	2.5 ounces	24	2.75	4.5	0
		818	49.25	138.5	10.25

MEAL #5

Food	Quantity	Calories	Protein	Carbs	Fat
Chicken breast	6 ounces	210	42	0	3.6
Rice	3.5 ounces	378	7	84	0.4
Green beans	2 ounces	19.2	1.2	4.1	0
		607.2	50.2	88.1	4.0

MEAL #6 (Postworkout)

Food	Quantity	Calories	Protein	Carbs	Fat
Oatmeal	3 ounces	351	12.6	61.2	6.6

3,300 CALORIES; APPROXIMATELY 25% PROTEIN, 65% CARBS, 10% FATS—TRADITIONAL BALANCE

DAY 6

MEAL #1

Food	Quantity	Calories	Protein	Carbs	Fat
Whole egg	1	80	6	0.6	5.6
Egg whites	7	112	24	2.9	0
Oatmeal	4 ounces	468	16.8	81.6	8.8
Nonfat milk	4 ounces	40	4	5.6	0.4
Banana	6 ounces	105	1.2	26.7	0.6
		805	52	117.4	15.4

MEAL #2

Food	Quantity	Calories	Protein	Carbs	Fat
Round steak	4.5 ounces	180	29.3	0	6.3
Lima beans	5.5 ounces	165	10	32	0
Rice	4 ounces	432	8	96	0.4
Spinach	3 ounces	23.2	3	4	0.4
		800.2	50.3	132	7.1

MEAL #3

Food	Quantity	Calories	Protein	Carbs	Fat
Turkey breast	5 ounces	175	35	0	3
Corn	10 ounces	280	10	65	3
Peas	10 ounces	220	16	38	1
Brussels sprouts	10 ounces	130	14	25	1
		805	75	128	8

MEAL #4

Food	Quantity	Calories	Protein	Carbs	Fat
Cod	3.5 ounces	80.5	18.6	0	0.35
Baked potato	15 ounces	342	9	76.5	0
Whole eggs	2	160	12	1.2	11.2
Asparagus	3 ounces	23.4	2.2	3.3	0
		605.9	41.8	81.0	11.55

MEAL #5 (Postworkout)

Food	Quantity	Calories	Protein	Carbs	Fat
Banana	16 ounces	280	3.2	71.2	1.6

3,000 CALORIES; APPROXIMATELY 55% PROTEIN, 35% CARBS, 10% FAT

DAY 7

MEAL #1

Food	Quantity	Calories	Protein	Carbs	Fat
Egg whites	12	192	40.8	5	0
Turkey breast	10 ounces	350	70	0	6
Oatmeal	1 ounce	117	4.2	20.4	2.2
Sweet potato	4 ounces	137	2.0	32	0.4
		796	117	57.4	8.6

MEAL #2

Food	Quantity	Calories	Protein	Carbs	Fat
Chicken breast	16 ounces	560	112	0	9.6
Rice	1 ounce	108	2	24	0.1
Broccoli	4 ounces	38.4	4.4	7.2	0
		706.4	118.4	31.2	9.7

MEAL #3

Food	Quantity	Calories	Protein	Carbs	Fat
Turkey breast	9 ounces	315	63	0	5.6
Lima beans	6 ounces	180	10.8	34.8	0
Peas	5 ounces	132	8	19	0.5
Spinach	3 ounces	23.4	3	3.9	0.3
		650.4	84.8	57.7	6.4

MEAL #4

Food	Quantity	Calories	Protein	Carbs	Fat
Red snapper	12 ounces	336	72	0	3.6
Rice	1.5 ounces	162	3	36	0.15
Green beans	6 ounces	57.6	3.6	12.6	0
		555.6	78.6	48.6	3.75

MEAL #5 (Postworkout)

Food	Quantity	Calories	Protein	Carbs	Fat
Sweet potato	8.5 ounces	290	4.25	68	0.85

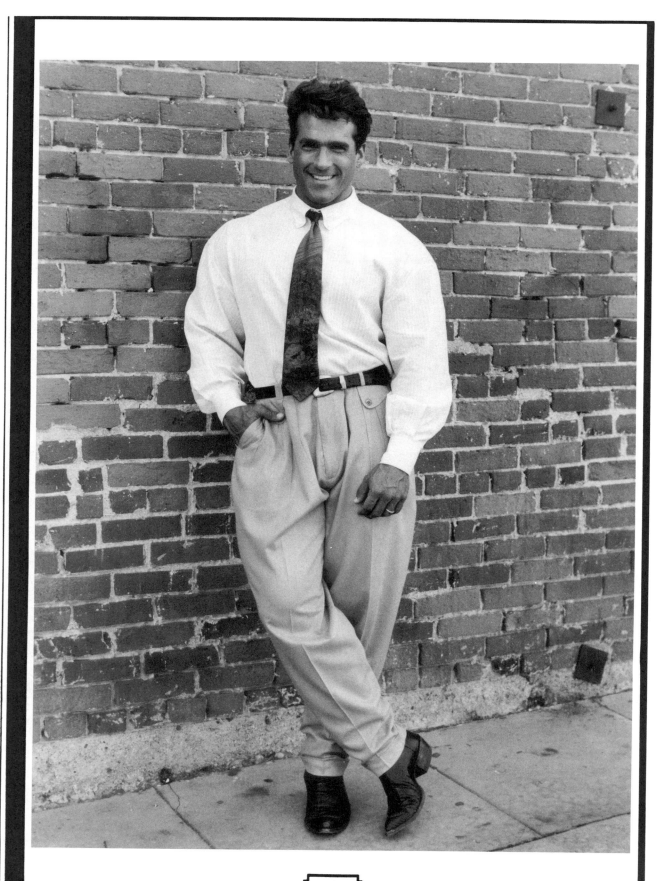

LOOKING GOOD

At the beginning of the book, I asked you to imagine that you were ten years old again and that this adventure represented your birthday and Christmas all rolled up into one giant ball of anticipation.

This section talks about some of the gift wrap on the surface of the presents you'll give yourself as you work toward looking and feeling great. Because I work in the public eye, I have had to become somewhat of an amateur grooming expert. Over the years I've discovered and incorporated into my own lifestyle some basic tips related to skin care, hair care and clothing. Think of them as the finishing touches on your Flawlessness package. In these next few pages I'd like to share them with you.

I don't know about you, but I don't have the extra time, energy or patience to spend hours putting together a "look"; so I say, keep it simple. The only people I ever hear say otherwise usually have expensive products to sell. Not that you shouldn't sometimes pamper yourself. For example, after a long, hard, stressful workday, I'll sometimes take a "mini vacation" by drawing a hot bath, getting in, soaking and letting my mind and body just unwind. A half hour later I'll feel relaxed and recharged. It may seem small and simple, but for me it works magic.

Here are some of my recommendations for keeping yourself looking great:

1. Develop a basic daily skin care routine. In my personal program, the first step is cleansing. I use a cleanser that is designed for my skin type. I'll wash

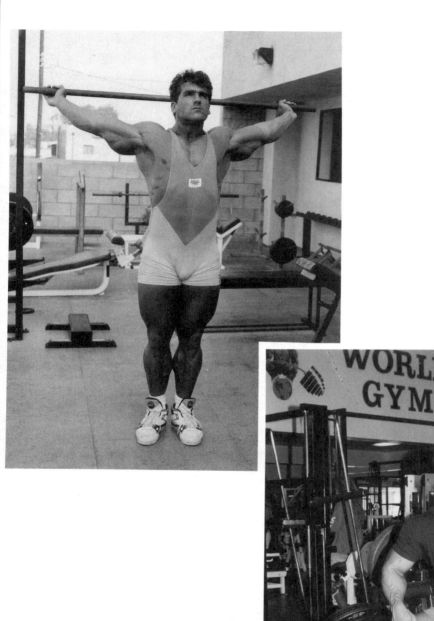

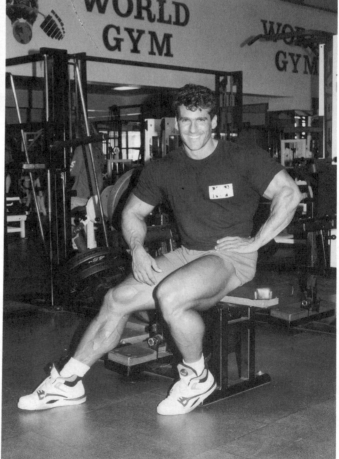

and rinse my entire face and neck, moving my fingertips in circular motions and really concentrating on areas where pores could get plugged.

Next I use a toner that hydrates the skin. I'll either wipe it on with a cotton ball or put it in a spray bottle and mist it on. Then, while my face is still wet with toner, I'll use a small amount of moisturizer. Because my face is still moist, I'll only need a very tiny amount. These three steps make up my daily routine and I use it twice a day, morning and night.

Once a week I use a light facial scrub to remove dead skin cells and make everything look fresh. I'm really careful not to overscrub my face, though, since skin gets irritated very easily.

As far as products are concerned, I look for simplicity and quality. The brands that I'd currently recommend are manufactured by a West Coast company called Garden Botanika. At present I have no financial ties to this company. I recommend it simply because I like its products. To order a product list, call (800) 877-9603, or write the company at 15510 Northeast 90th Street, Redmond, Washington, 98052.

2. Moisturize your body. This is really important year-round to keep your skin elastic and young looking. You should put on moisturizer immediately after a bath or shower, when your skin is still partially wet. Since moisturizer is used to trap water against the skin, its use on dry skin is not nearly as effective. I'd also recommend the Garden Botanika skin moisturizers.

3. If you tan, always do so cautiously. I don't need to tell you about the dangers of overexposure to the sun and the direct link between tanning and skin cancer. Build your exposure up slowly, because every major sunburn you get exponentially increases your chances of skin cancer later in life. If you must work or play in the sun, use a strong sunscreen and reapply it hourly if you sweat or go in the water. Use a skin moisturizer with aloe vera to hydrate tanned skin.

4. Find a good hairstylist and get a haircut that blends with the shape of your face. Also, use high-quality shampoos and conditioners. When you find a stylist, talk about what you want your hair to look like *before* any cutting takes place. You should also find out how much maintenance will be involved in getting the hair back to the look you leave the salon with.

I like to rotate shampoos so that my hair doesn't get used to any one kind. I keep three different types and use a different one each time I shower. I use a conditioner on my hair once a week. Consult your stylist about your individual needs.

5. If you aren't a clotheshorse, try to build a basic, interchangeable wardrobe that fits not only your body, but your work and social needs.

I like my clothes to fit well, but kind of loose. My feeling is that I don't have to show my body off everywhere I go. For the most part, I dress casually and buy most of my clothes at retail stores like The Gap, Banana Republic and Eddie Bauer. All these stores have clothes that are oversized and very well made. They also all have a very good return policy if you get home and something isn't quite up to your standards. Eddie Bauer, I should note, has a very fast catalogue service and recently added XXL shirt sizes in nearly all of its styles.

Keep your clothing investment looking great by following the washing or dry-cleaning instructions on the garment label.

Here are a few "luxury items" that you can consider for yourself—especially if you're using your Flawless program to build up to a big event, like a reunion, where you really want to look your best. Go ahead and indulge yourself.

1. **Have a new outfit (or two) tailor-made to fit your body perfectly.**
2. **Get a complete facial.**
3. **Get a manicure and/or pedicure.**
4. **Get a full-body sports massage.**
5. **Work with a color consultant who'll match your hair and skin tones with the best clothing colors.**
6. **Take a twenty-minute nap every day. It will do wonders for the bags under your eyes.**
7. **Take the time to remind yourself that you deserve to have a great body, perfect health and self-respect.**

INDEX

Reverse-grip push-downs, 190, 196
Reverse pec-decks, 79
Reverse push-downs, 220, 230
Rope extensions, 238, 247
Rope push-downs, 175, 184, 214, 224
Rotation exercises, 23–24
Rowing movement, 22–23, 73–74

Scissors, 65; apprentice, 136, 141, 146, 150, 155; journeyman, 189, 195, 220, 230; master, 192, 205
Seated barbell presses behind neck, 203, 212
Seated bent-over side raises: journeyman, 172, 182, 190, 196, 203, 212, 239, 247; master, 175, 184
Seated calf raise, 63, 93; apprentice, 136, 141, 146, 150, 155, 161; journeyman, 172, 181, 189, 190, 196, 203, 204, 213, 214, 222, 230, 247; master, 174, 175, 183, 184, 197, 205, 215, 225, 231, 232, 240, 241
Seated dumbbell presses: journeyman, 172, 182, 189, 195; master, 191, 297, 206, 215, 249
Seated dumbbell side raises: journeyman, 203, 212; master, 192, 205
Seated French presses: journeyman, 220, 230; master, 248
Seated machine leg curls, 90
Seated presses behind back: journeyman, 189, 196; master, 214, 224
Secondary muscles, 18
Self-evaluation, 131–32, 199–200
Self-inspection, 121–22
Self-massage, 123, 210
Self-therapy, 210–11
Shoulder presses, 30–32
Shoulder rotation movement, 73–75
Shoulders: how they work, 29–32; movement exercises for, 79–82; positioning, 19
Shrug movements, 73, 76–77
Single-arm cable curl, 24
Sissy squats, 87, 88; master, 197, 205, 232, 241
Soreness, treatment of, 210
Sport-specific, 98
Squat, 32, 243–44
Stair-climbing machine, 107

Standing alternating dumbbell curls, 197, 205, 215, 249
Standing calf raises, 62, 98; apprentice, 120, 125, 130, 136, 141, 146, 150, 156, 161; journeyman, 172, 181, 189, 196, 204, 214, 222, 231, 247; master, 174, 183, 197, 205, 206, 216, 231, 240, 249, 250
Standing leg curls, 90; journeyman, 173, 182, 189, 195, 203, 213, 222, 230, 239, 247, 248; master, 175, 184, 191, 198, 206, 216, 231, 240, 249, 250
Stationary bicycle, 106
Stiff-leg deadlifts, 34–35, 36, 73, 78, 90–91; journeyman, 204, 214, 222, 231, 247; master, 174, 183, 197, 205, 206, 215, 216, 225, 232, 241, 250
Straight-arm pull-ins, 23, 73, 74–75; master, 197, 205, 207, 215, 224, 241
Stretch position, 16–17, 43, 98, 99–103
Stretching and aerobics, 95–108
Stretching movements, 90–91
Super-set, 228
Supination, 24
Supplements, 115, 179–81

Target heart rate, 105
T-bar rows, 73, 74; journeyman, 190, 196, 222, 231; master, 176, 197, 205, 231, 240
Tibia movements, 93, 94
Tibia raises, 174, 175, 183, 184, 197, 198, 205, 206, 215, 216, 225, 231, 232, 240, 241, 249, 250
Training: apprentice, 114–15, 118, 122–23, 128–29, 134, 138–39, 143–44, 148, 152–53, 159; journeyman/ master, 167–68, 178–79, 186, 193–94, 203–4, 210–11, 218, 243–45
Triceps, 84–86; how they work, 26–29
Triceps-pressing exercises, 26
Triceps push-downs, 28–29, 57, 116, 125, 130
Tri-sets, 228
Two-arm, one-dumbbell extensions, 214, 224
Two-arm dumbbell rows, 73
Two-arm preacher curls, 225, 233
Two-arm pulley curls, 83, 233
Two-arm pulley preacher curls, 83
Two-arm pulley rows, 225

Two-arm pulley wrist curls, 91
Two-arm reverse-pulley wrist curls, 91
Two-dumbbell kickbacks: journeyman, 189, 195, 204, 213; master, 174, 183, 206, 215, 232, 241, 249
Two-dumbbell rows, 241
Two-dumbbell wrist curls: journeyman, 189, 195, 203, 213, 247; master, 197, 206, 207, 224, 241
Two-pulley rear crunches, 214, 224, 248
Twisting crunches: journeyman, 190, 196, 222, 231; master, 175, 184, 192, 205, 225, 240, 249

Underhanded pull-ups, 24
Upright rows, 79, 80, 81; journeyman, 172, 182, 204, 213, 238, 247; master, 225, 239, 248

Valine, 188
Variation, 44
Variety, 167
Vegetables, fibrous, 236
Visualization, 3

Weight drops, 214
Weighted side bends, 40
Wide front pull-downs, 48, 49, 73; journeyman, 181, 203, 213, 222, 231, 239, 248; master, 197, 205, 215, 241, 249
Wide front pull-ups, 73, 191, 198, 215, 230, 249
Wide-grip low-pulley row, 231, 240
Wide-grip pull-downs, 175, 183, 190
Wide-grip rear pull-downs, 48, 73; journeyman, 189, 195, 204, 214; master, 176, 191, 198, 207, 224, 225, 232
Wide rear pull-ups, 73, 197, 205, 247
Workouts: types of, 104–5; volume of, 186. *See also* Training
Wrist-curling movements, 91, 93

Zottman curls, 91–93, 176, 197, 206, 225, 233, 241